# Praise for *The Ayurvedic Approach to Cancer*

'Dr Sam Watts has beautifully woven together the ancient wisdom of Ayurveda with the modern realities of cancer care in this thought-provoking and empowering book. His focus on engaging the body's healing potential through mindset, immune support and alignment with chronobiological systems deeply resonates with my own work, especially his emphasis on survivorship and the holistic balance of the terrain. I am particularly impressed by his keen insights into patient empowerment and pattern recognition – a hallmark of Ayurveda that has stood the test of time.

'While our approaches to dietary recommendations may differ, particularly in how we address the metabolic aspects of cancer treatment, I wholeheartedly support his overarching philosophy of nurturing the whole being. Dr Watts' 5-Step Plan to mitigate side effects and enhance wellbeing will undoubtedly offer readers a comprehensive and holistic path to health. His deep understanding of the profound role that ancient herbal medicines can play in cancer care is a valuable contribution to the ongoing conversation about integrative oncology.'

NASHA WINTERS, ND, FABNO, coauthor of *The Metabolic Approach to Cancer* and *Mistletoe and the Emerging Future of Integrative Oncology*

'*The Ayurvedic Approach to Cancer* is among the next generation of required reading for patients and healthcare providers. Cancer rates have surpassed pandemic levels, and this book delivers significant scientific pushback against these unacceptable trends using the effective and time-tested framework of Ayurvedic medicine. Dr Watts provides requisite emphasis on psychology, offers a refreshing food-forward focus and describes powerful sensory-driven healing modalities. Bring a highlighter – the content is both life-changing and easy to digest.'

JESS HIGGINS KELLEY, MNT, ONC, founder and director of the Oncology Nutrition Institute and coauthor of *The Metabolic Approach to Cancer*

'In this outstanding book, Dr Sam Watts explores ways to unlock your body's innate power to heal with the time-tested principles of Ayurveda and groundbreaking insights from exceptional cancer survivorship research. Dr Watts combines his expertise in Ayurvedic medicine with a PhD in cancer survivorship to offer a practical, evidence-based guide for those seeking holistic support. From anti-cancer nutrition and herbal medicine to mindset shifts and sensory healing, this transformative book empowers readers with a step-by-step plan to harness their full potential in the face of a cancer diagnosis. Here at The Complementary Medical Association (The CMA), we unreservedly recommend this book to practitioners – and people living with cancer.'

JAYNEY GODDARD, president of The Complementary Medical Association

# The Ayurvedic Approach to Cancer

# The Ayurvedic Approach to Cancer

Engaging your body's
powerful healing abilities
through mindset, diet
and lifestyle

**Dr Sam Watts**
**Foreword by Jasmine Hemsley**
**Introduction by Robin Daly**

Chelsea Green Publishing
London, UK
White River Junction, Vermont, USA

First published in 2025 by Chelsea Green Publishing | PO Box 4529 | White River Junction, VT 05001 |
West Wing, Somerset House, Strand | London, WC2R 1LA, UK | www.chelseagreen.com
A Division of Rizzoli International Publications, Inc. | 49 West 27th Street | New York, NY 10001 | www.rizzoliusa.com
Gruppo Mondadori | Via privata Mondadori, 1 | 20054 Segrate (Milano), ITA

Copyright © 2025 by Sam Watts.
All rights reserved.

Unless otherwise noted, all illustrations copyright © 2025 by Sam Watts.

No part of this book may be transmitted or reproduced in any form by any means without permission in writing from the publisher.

**Disclaimer:** This book is designed to provide helpful information on the subjects discussed. It is not meant to be used, nor should it be used, to diagnose or treat any medical condition without the supervision of an appropriate medical professional or doctor. For diagnosis or treatment of any medical problem, please consult your own physician or a suitable professional practitioner. The publisher and author are not liable for any damages or negative consequences from any treatment, action, application or preparation to any person reading or following the information in this book. References are provided for informational purposes only and do not constitute endorsement of any websites or sources. Readers should be aware that the websites listed in this book may change. The information and references included are up to date at the time of writing but given that medical evidence progresses, they may not be up to date at the time of reading. Personal names given in case histories have been changed to preserve privacy/anonymity.

Publisher: Charles Miers
Deputy Publisher: Matthew Derr
Commissioning Editor: Muna Reyal
Project Manager: Susan Pegg
Copy Editor: Susan Pegg
Proofreader: Jacqui Lewis
Indexer: Charmian Parkin
Designer: Melissa Jacobson
Page Layout: Jenna Richardson

ISBN 978-1-915294-48-7 (paperback) | ISBN 978-1-915294-49-4 (ebook) | ISBN 978-1-915294-50-0 (audiobook)
Library of Congress Control Number: 2024045824 (print)
A CIP catalogue record for this book is available from the British Library.

**Our Commitment to Green Publishing**
Chelsea Green sees publishing as a tool for cultural change and ecological stewardship. We strive to align our book manufacturing practices with our editorial mission and to reduce the impact of our business enterprise in the environment. We print our books using vegetable-based inks whenever possible. This book may cost slightly more because it was printed on paper from responsibly managed forests, and we hope you'll agree that it's worth it. *The Ayurvedic Approach to Cancer* was printed on paper supplied by Lake Book Manufacturing that is made of recycled materials and other controlled sources.

Authorized EU representative for product safety and compliance
Mondadori Libri S.p.A. | www.mondadori.it
via Gian Battista Vico 42 | Milan, Italy 20123

Printed in the United States of America.
10 9 8 7 6 5 4 3 2 1     25 26 27 28 29

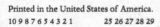
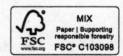

*This book is dedicated to my three amazing children, Xavier, Trixie and Xanthe. Always live brightly, my little ones.*

*And to my beautiful wife, Holly; with love, forever.*

# Contents

| | |
|---|---|
| *Foreword by Jasmine Hemsley* | *xi* |
| *Introduction by Robin Daly* | *xiii* |
| 1. The Insanity of Impossible | 1 |
| 2. Choosing Your Own Reality | 9 |
| 3. The Biology of Hope | |
|    *Unlocking the Gates of Exceptional* | 25 |
| 4. Onwards to Imagery | |
|    *The Recreation of Reality* | 47 |
| 5. Laying Strong Foundations | |
|    *Ayurvedic Anti-Cancer Nutrition* | 63 |
| 6. Agni and Ojas | |
|    *The Elixir of Health and Immunity* | 93 |
| 7. Nature's Pharmacy | |
|    *Anti-Cancer Herbal Medicines* | 119 |
| 8. Dancing to Nature's Rhythm | |
|    *Chronobiology and the New Frontier of Cancer Survivorship* | 139 |
| 9. Awakening the Body's Inner Pharmacy | |
|    *The Sensory Pathways of Healing* | 165 |
| 10. Putting Out the Fires | |
|    *Managing the Side Effects of Conventional Cancer Treatments* | 187 |
| 11. Bringing It All Together | |
|    *The 5-Step Plan* | 201 |
| Conclusion | 213 |
| *Acknowledgements* | *217* |
| *Appendix 1: Vikruti Assessment Questionnaire* | *219* |
| *Appendix 2: Envisioning Health* | *223* |
| *Appendix 3: Ayurvedic and Herbal Suppliers* | *227* |
| *Glossary* | *229* |
| *Notes* | *231* |
| *Index* | *245* |

# Foreword

This book begins with a story about acid reflux, which immediately resonated with me. My own journey to Ayurveda began over twenty years ago, when I was seeking an alternative to healing this 'normalised condition' and avoiding the higher-strength antacids I was being prescribed.

As someone whose job it was to 'look' healthy (I was a professional model at the time), I thought I was living a 'healthy lifestyle' by exercising and eating well, but I soon discovered through Ayurveda that our health is much more nuanced than this. (I hope this sounds intriguing... You'll find out what I mean soon enough in this book!) Thankfully, I trusted my intuition to look to a holistic alternative to treat the cause of my ailment rather than just continue to mask the symptoms. Only a few days into using a basic Ayurvedic remedy, my reflux was gone and, as I integrated my new learnings with some shifts to my eating behaviour, it never returned. It was simple, felt instinctively right and my body responded quickly. I was hooked, and I have spent the last twenty years absorbing Ayurvedic wisdom practices, weaving them into the framework of my life and helping others to integrate them too.

Discovering Dr Sam Watts' informative insights into the wonders of Ayurveda via Instagram was a breath of fresh air for me, as well as a sigh of relief – here was a Western-trained cancer researcher providing authentic Ayurvedic traditions in an accessible way. By combining thousands of years of tried-and-tested Eastern wisdom with the latest medical advances for contemporary needs, Dr Sam's book helps give a balanced view on all the information available. The practices of Ayurveda have become part of my everyday routine – supporting my mental, emotional and physical wellbeing and positively influencing those around me. However, there is the notion outside alternative communities – and maybe even within them – that when it comes to serious disease, and especially 'the big C', there is no room for 'alternative medicine' in modern healthcare and a more direct and aggressive approach is needed. The irony is that there is not a more direct approach than going to the root cause of the health issue by using a holistic approach that is thorough, bespoke to the individual and usually minimally invasive – a win-win-win.

I found *The Ayurvedic Approach to Cancer* an engaging read, filled with well-explained Ayurvedic wisdom and easy-to-implement practices. On hearing the title of this book, I felt very emotional and reading it has been particularly poignant. My dad was diagnosed with cancer three times over a fifteen-year period, and sadly the third time it played a role in his death. My experience during this time led me to believe that a complete and drastic reframing of health and healing is very much needed. I wish this book had been available when we were looking for ways to support him, especially during the last diagnosis when he showed an interest in non-conventional avenues but was already weak and overwhelmed. The fusion of Ayurveda with Western science and clinical studies would have no doubt given my dad (a no-nonsense military man of action) a framework to explore alternative ideas of health that could have supported his physical and mental wellbeing during his long, drawn-out illness.

Over the course of my health and wellbeing journey, from writing my own book on Ayurveda to working with and experiencing first-hand the incredible community of Ayurvedic doctors (*vaidyas*) and practitioners, I am both relieved and inspired at how Ayurveda has become more mainstream and accepted as a proven system of health. I truly hope that Dr Sam's new book will be embraced and continue to bring Ayurvedic wisdom to a wider audience – something that is clearly needed in the face of an alarming global rise of chronic disease and, indeed, cancer.

For those out there who want to have autonomy over their own health and play an active part in their health journey, whether facing a prognosis or not, this manual can help them and their doctors better understand that there is more to health than what the current medical system offers. That the complementary medicine of Ayurveda can meet them where they are at and support them holistically, whichever route they choose to take. My hope is that we can soon reach a time where a holistic approach is no longer niche and an integrated health system is the standard and available to everyone. I am convinced more than ever that when we work with nature, deep and profound healing is possible and the prevention of disease is better managed – imagine the boon to our healthcare system if we were educated and empowered on a natural approach to our wellbeing! With this book, you have an expert in your corner who understands both the holistic and mainstream medical world. I hope that this book gives us the next big breakthrough we need. Thank you, Dr Sam, for this book.

JASMINE HEMSLEY, author of *East by West*, chef and wellbeing expert

# Introduction

Dr Sam Watts is an important voice for our times. He is an inspirational and visionary leader in health and wellbeing, whose message of hope and positivity is both welcome and urgently needed.

Sam is the embodiment of the synthesis that this brilliant new book represents: science and tradition, East and West, the why and the how. After decades of focusing on the cellular biochemistry of human bodies and how we can influence this with chemical interventions, Western science has begun to give attention to understanding the forces that support wellbeing and innate healing. These turn out to be both outer and inner – behaviours and environments, as well as thoughts and feelings. In fact, *The Ayurvedic Approach to Cancer* makes the case for the foundational role our perspective on life has in directing the course of our physical and mental wellbeing – particularly when faced with an existential challenge such as cancer.

Over and above knowledge about specific diseases and conditions, what Ayurveda possesses is a deep understanding of health, of the elements of wellbeing. This enables it to address a problem as formidable as cancer at the foundational level – a critical step for lasting success to become a possibility. Ayurvedic practice acknowledges the central role of meaning and purpose in a life, and here we are touching on the mystery of what life really is: what is that light that once snuffed out leaves behind an empty shell, a corpse devoid of the person we knew? That light is the very force of life itself and the will to live in action; it is a manifestation of meaning and purpose, and of hope expressed in time.

Right at the heart of the book, in the chapter Laying Strong Foundations, Sam delivers a clear expression of the radical 'East meets West' synthesis that he is leading. The seven hallmarks of cancer, which are so clearly explained in this book, represent the most universally recognised descriptions of the unique characteristics of the disease. They are used by pharmaceutical companies the world over to identify therapeutic targets and develop treatments. Here, Sam uses them in exactly the same manner, only instead to identify dietary interventions based on Ayurvedic principles. He shows us the clinical evidence around the ability of specific foods to suppress these primary hallmarks, which are so instrumental in the way cancer grows and spreads.

Sam is a researcher with a thirst for understanding the mechanisms of health. But he is also one of those rare scientists with an appreciation that while, on the one hand, we're never going to be able to explain all the mysteries of life through biochemistry alone, on the other, it is critical that we have observed experimental data to show us the way. What might have been common sense or intuitive in past times is either no longer available to us or seen as trustworthy. This is where what I call 'the science of the obvious' is desperately needed: a clear scientific demonstration of the fact that following common sense, intuition or 'inner wisdom' makes complete sense. The science that has predominated in this field is psychoneuroimmunology, or PNI, and its progress over the last thirty years or so is a story of steadily mounting evidence of the absolute inseparability of mind and body. This is the premise of everything that Sam has to offer in his advocacy of, and leadership in, what is now commonly described as 'mind-body medicine'. We owe much to courageous researchers such as Sam for their willingness plunge into the less tangible realms of survivorship; to establish for all our sakes what the truth is about the factors that most significantly influence our ability to recover.

Sam describes Ayurveda as the science of optimal living, and it is sobering to witness how the immense investment in PNI research merely underpins what was already understood and documented thousands of years ago. Alongside this development, practices that form essential elements of Ayurveda, and that just a few decades ago were distinctly 'foreign', have since made inroads into Western life in ways that would previously have been unthinkable. It's hugely encouraging that meditation and mindfulness are now common currency in education, business and even politics, and yoga is a regular practice that is unlikely to raise eyebrows.

Above all, the direction that Ayurveda points is towards living in a way that is 'connected', ultimately towards 'oneness'. Since the malaise of the twenty-first century could well be described in terms of disconnectedness, this ideally places Ayurveda to help address our current needs. Despite being more connected, digitally, than ever before, we are perilously disconnected from our bodies, from our intuition, from one other and from our environment. We are experiencing a collective crisis of trust, preferring increasingly to live in artificial environments created by humans that feed our desires while numbing our consciousness and starving our souls. Unsurprisingly, this is resulting in a chaotic descent into chronic ill health – including cancer, a disease characterised by the development of cells suffering from an eerily parallel disconnectedness from the broader environment and wholesome purpose of the body.

In my work with Yes to Life, I share with Sam the experience of repeatedly meeting people who had been predicted to die but simply had not. They had reached a point where they had decided it wasn't 'their time', reclaimed their autonomy and took charge of their situation in some way – so many different ways, in fact, that the common factors seem to be less about the 'what' than about the 'how' of their approaches. Western medicine has largely bypassed one of the most important factors affecting lives and lifespans – the will to live. This irrepressibly positive force is fed primarily by the very factors that society has been leading us rapidly away from: connection to others and to our environment. It is the source of our passions in life and is inextricably bound up with hope – which is why it is so critical to respect and nurture hope in those we aim to support.

Sam embodies all the very best aspects of a medical carer, as set out in the aspirational 'Yes to Life Charter for Oncology', and it is a privilege to collaborate with him regularly. First and foremost, he is a living example of his message, a radically positive expression of Life, deeply engaged in positive action to help as many as possible; secondly, as a scientist and practitioner, he is well informed and highly skilled; thirdly, he is open-minded in his embrace of everything from the technical to the esoteric.

*The Ayurvedic Approach to Cancer* makes a hugely supportive contribution to the arena, and I am in no doubt that it will be a 'lifesaver' for many, opening up a possible, even an exciting, future from their impossible predicament. It addresses both the 'why' and the 'how' amply, with explanations of the biochemistry rubbing shoulders with Ayurvedic recipes. There is a wealth of practical advice on important topics, such as meeting the side effects of conventional treatments with tried and trusted natural approaches.

Ultimately, this book and, indeed, the entire focus of Sam's life and work is Love. This is what drives him, what gets him out of bed in the morning, and is the fuel for the radical transformations he is inspiring in those he supports.

ROBIN DALY, founder and chairman of Yes to Life,
the UK's integrative cancer care charity

# CHAPTER ONE

# The Insanity of Impossible

> *And those who were seen to be dancing were thought to be insane by those who could not hear the music.*
>
> OLD PROVERB

Janet was a healthy, happy and vibrant sixty-one-year-old with much to be grateful for and much to look forward to. Her three grown-up children were settled in loving relationships with good jobs and happy lives. Her own life was just as happy; she was approaching her thirtieth wedding anniversary to her childhood sweetheart, whom she loved more with each passing year. She had recently moved into semi-retirement, which had given her more time to engage in her passions and interests – music, learning to paint, photography and, most of all, travel. And with full retirement not far off, she was joyous in her anticipation of the unique opportunities that a well-planned-for retirement can offer to someone who has worked hard for it.

Janet also felt blessed to be vibrantly well, full of energy and in all regards a picture of health. Indeed, other than for a few niggling and relatively insignificant symptoms, Janet rated her health as being better now than it had been ten years ago when she was working long hours in a stressful finance position. However, one of those niggling little symptoms that just wouldn't go away was heartburn, something that Janet had infrequently suffered with for many years. So when it started occurring a little more often, she thought nothing of it. But as the weeks went by, the niggle became more of a noticeable nuisance that began needing more management. She would periodically find herself going to bed propped up on pillows to help alleviate the heartburn. She was buying and using over-the-counter antacids on a weekly basis, and after a month or so the acid reflux began to directly impact upon what she could and couldn't eat.

At this point, Janet still thought nothing was too amiss because of how well she felt in herself. Nevertheless, she decided to visit her doctor just to be sure, which resulted in a referral for an endoscopy at the local hospital so that a clearer diagnosis could be gleaned. And while she was aware that she was being fast-tracked through the system, none of the medical professionals she encountered thought anything particularly sinister was going on; chronic acid reflux or GORD (gastro-oesophageal reflux disorder) was an incredibly common ailment, which the doctors assessing her said they saw every week.

But then came the bombshell. Janet didn't have GORD. She had a very aggressive and established stage 3 stomach cancer, which had migrated into her oesophagus. The next few weeks were a blur: tests, scans, appointments, fear, uncertainty and compounding bad news. Eventually, Janet's treatment regime was confirmed and she commenced an aggressive eight-week cycle of chemotherapy to help shrink the tumour. This was followed by a hugely invasive surgery in which over half of her stomach was removed. She then completed another gruelling eight-week cycle of chemotherapy just to be sure that any cancer cells missed by the surgery were destroyed.

After such a punishing series of treatments, Janet began the slow process of proactively rebuilding her strength and her health. And over the next year, her quarterly scans and follow-ups brought progressively good news: no cancer recurrence and good blood markers. But one cold and rainy November afternoon, the ground opened up once again. The cancer had returned and now a large fist-sized tumour was wrapped around a rich and complex network of blood vessels in her abdominal cavity, rendering it inoperable. It was aggressive, fast growing and incurable. The only treatment options available were palliative rather than curative and a ten-week cycle of targeted radiotherapy was decided upon. This was to help contain the spread of the cancer and hopefully provide a little more time for Janet; this was the best that could be hoped for.

In the face of the utter hopelessness of her situation, Janet found herself lost, depressed and scared. But as is so often the case, the darkest places are where we find the greatest inspiration. With immense inner fortitude, Janet slowly regrouped, refocused and began to reperceive her position. Upon doing so, she decided there and then to bring a completely different reality to bear on the situation she was facing.

Unwilling to accept the script put in front of her and the tyranny of the statistics she had been offered, she point-blank refused to let the incurable prognosis she had been given railroad her onto a path that, in her mind, wasn't hers to follow. Even more so, she unequivocally refused to allow this cancer to threaten everything she was so desperate to live for: her husband, her children and her grandchildren; her music, art and photography; her planned travels around the world, the deserted beaches, ice-bound fjords and the world's most famous museums and galleries from which she drew immense energy and inspiration.

So, she decided that her best option was not to try to rewrite the impossibly negative script handed to her but rather to write her own script. This was a script that offered health, longevity, hope, love and, ultimately, a future. This was an outright refusal to allow the oppressive negativity that surrounded every part of her prognosis to hijack her dreams, her beliefs and her very life.

Ultimately, Janet did the only thing that was available to her: she retook control. She began researching her options, opened her mind to new opportunities and ultimately decided that to be successful in her pursuit of the impossible, adopting a few simple dietary and lifestyle changes (as important as these are) would not be enough. Not by a long way. Rather, what was needed was a complete restructuring of the very fabric of her existence. She intuitively knew that she would need to approach her health, her healing and her very consciousness through a completely different lens that was operating within a wildly different rubric of understanding if she was to succeed. Remembering a line from a book she had recently read, she realised this was not about thinking outside of the box but rather removing the restraints of the box altogether.

As a close family member of mine, Janet was well versed in the world of natural medicine and so she turned to the integrative, time-tested and evidence-based healing modalities of Ayurveda. And within the healing embrace of this most exceptional of medical systems, Janet found something that was truly vital in her quest for survival: empowerment.

She discovered within the wisdom traditions of Ayurveda an entire blueprint for complete and total health transformation, in both mind and body. This blueprint was documented, evidence-based and time-tested; it just needed to be picked up, adopted and run with. And so Janet ran. Doing so not only provided her with a clear focus of what she needed to do to reclaim her health but how to actually go about doing so. That very singular act of empowerment changed the entire inner dialogue operating within Janet's mind: hopelessness was transformed into hope, helplessness into action, fear into confidence and impossible into possible.

Over the coming months, she began to slowly, progressively and robustly adopt an entirely new framework of being, seeing and existing in the world that was guided by the ancient healing traditions of Ayurveda. This framework impacted upon every part of herself. Not just the obvious aspects of what we associate with healing, such as diet, exercise and stress reduction, but also the identification and activation of the subtler and therefore more profound aspects of healing – the elevation of consciousness, the cultivation of transformational belief systems and moving into a life fuelled by the Vedic concept of *dharma*, which equates to a life filled with meaning, purpose and passion.

Then, slowly but consistently, things began to change. Her three-monthly scans showed that the growth of her tumours had slowed down. And then stopped. Then actually and impossibly shrunk. Very slowly, the dialogue with her oncologist also began to change. The first ripples of hope began to permeate the previously cold hopelessness of her clinical consultations. Even more importantly, the inner dialogue within Janet's mind changed. The tangible possibility of recovery and survival, something that had previously been purely hope and trust, suddenly broke through into the quantitative reality of her world.

Sixteen months after her terminal recurrence, Janet's oncologist called her into the hospital and opened up the discussion with these words: 'Today I am doing something that I have never done before and that my training has taught me is not possible. It is my absolute pleasure to declare someone with incurable stage 4 cancer as officially being in full remission.'

Janet's latest scan had, for the first time, revealed no visible signs of cancer. Not even microscopic levels. Today, just over five years later, Janet has been fully discharged from her oncology care team. She left a few very baffled and confused, but ultimately very happy, consultants and surgeons in her wake, all of whom were completely unable to account for her recovery. And this is as it should be. What accounted for Janet's exceptional survival was not something quantifiably and observably done 'to' her. Rather, what accounted for it was the seismic shift in her inner environment – her immune activity, her inflammatory pathways, her nutritional load and so much else besides – that ultimately allowed her body to unleash its unimaginably powerful inner pharmacy and bring this to bear on her cancer in a way that was simply irresistible.

But the key point is that this opportunity for becoming exceptional is not Janet's alone. It belongs to and exists within each and every one of us. Always and without exception. And with each passing year, more and more clinical research is adding to the existing foundation of evidence that shows just how powerful the human body's capacity for healing is. Even, and perhaps especially, in the face of terminal and incurable diseases.

It is this research that has ultimately led to the formation of a whole new discipline of scientific study in the field of oncology: that of the exceptional cancer patient. This paradigm-changing area of research concerns itself with the clinical investigation of individuals living with incurable and terminal cancers who defy the statistical odds facing them by going on to enjoy decades of health and in many cases full remission. What these exceptional individuals achieve is, clinically and conventionally speaking, impossible in a similar way to how Janet's recovery was. And yet the science clearly and unequivocally shows us that it is possible, and every year the foundation of clinical evidence supporting what accounts for such exceptional cancer survival grows stronger. The rationale underpinning this area of research is that if it's possible to find consistent commonalities that the majority of exceptional cancer patients adopt into their lives, it would be highly likely that these commonalities accounted for what allowed them to become exceptional in the first place. Such consistencies have now been found to exist and the vast majority of them fall under the framework of Ayurveda, a holistic system of medicine that originated in India over five thousand years ago.

The aim of this book is to marry together the two unique and independent areas of exceptional cancer survivorship research and Ayurveda into a unified, practical and easy-to-follow blueprint that you can adopt into your life and through doing so transform it. Ultimately, my hope is that this book will inspire you to strive for the exceptional and believe in the impossible while showing you how Ayurveda can help you to get there. Not as an alternative to or replacement for conventional cancer treatments but as an adjunct to it; not to explore, discuss and benefit from the proven cancer treatments available within the field of conventional medicine would be as much of a mistake as not exploring the profound healing benefits of Ayurveda. After all, when we divide, we always weaken. Surely the best model for becoming exceptional in the face of a cancer diagnosis is a deeply holistic one. This is a model that sees us integrate all the best available practices from both West and East into a singular unified model of healing. Doing so maximises our ability to unleash the full possibility of becoming exceptional in the most effective way possible.

Helping, encouraging and guiding as many people as possible to achieve this is my profession, my passion and in many ways my obsession. Looking back, I can see that this has very much been the case since my formative years. For when I was growing up in London as a young boy, a new neighbour called Adrian moved into our road who turned out to be a Sri Lankan clinician trained in both Western and Eastern medicine, including homeopathy and Ayurveda. When my family and I fell ill with common household ailments, coughs and colds, it was to Adrian we turned and, as the years went by, he became a close and trusted family friend. To this day, I owe a true debt of gratitude to this inspirational man; he first lit the spark of my interest in all things healing and natural medicine. The limitless potential for healing that was to be found in the subtle intricacies of the human body and how to mobilise this healing in the face of disease was as mesmerising as it was captivating. These views ultimately went on to shape my own and they awakened in me a profound desire to help people that eventually led to me establishing a career in clinical cancer research at the University of Southampton School of Medicine.

It was there that I gained my PhD, studying cancer survivorship mechanisms in men with prostate cancer. The driving question that guided every aspect of my research was: 'How can I help people with cancer to actually and tangibly thrive – physically and emotionally – when living with their diagnosis?' In other words, how could I establish an evidence-based model that would help overcome the endemic levels of suffering, anxiety, depression and fear that are so commonplace in those living with cancer and replace these with their diametric opposites: hope, positivity, empowerment, optimism and self-belief? For as we shall explore as we move through this book, cultivating these types of mindsets is absolutely vital in the pursuit of exceptional cancer survivorship.

In answering this question, my passion and background in the Eastern tradition of healing merged with my training in the world of conventional cancer research as I began to scientifically test the impacts and efficacy of mind-body practices such as meditation. The results were hugely encouraging, showing that these practices were clinically effective at reducing emotional suffering, anxiety and depression while also helping to optimise physical health and wellbeing in those living with cancer. This very much fuelled the fire in me to further explore such practices so as to validate their integration and adoption into the Western arena of integrative cancer care.

To facilitate this, I was awarded a National Institute for Health Research Fellowship that afforded me the opportunity to develop, run and contribute to a variety of different clinical trials and studies within the field of integrative cancer research at a selection of different National Health Service hospitals in London and South East England. Over time, this research evolved to explore how mind-body practices could positively modulate not only psychological variables but also immunological, physiological and genetic ones. I immersed myself in this world and became obsessed with reading and studying every single piece of clinical research I could access around understanding the clinical, immunological, psychological and behavioural variables that were predictive of better survivorship outcomes in those living with cancer, particularly with regard to the exceptional cancer survivors to whom we have previously referred.

It was also during this time that I was blessed to meet Professor George Lewith, who would go on to become the most influential mentor of my professional life and powerfully shape my subsequent career trajectory and passions. This exceptional professor was a truly pioneering clinician with a passion for natural medicine and for over a decade he tirelessly schooled me in the foundations of complementary and integrative medicine. Under his tutorage I immersed myself in these worlds and embarked on an immersive study of Ayurveda and herbal medicine.

Slowly, over time, I began to integrate the foundational concepts and teachings of these disciplines into the cancer survivorship programmes I was running while simultaneously immersing myself in the clinical trial data exploring the evidence base for doing so. Then, the stars aligned and I experienced a powerful eureka moment as I saw, with profound clarity, the full and unparalleled potential of integrating Ayurveda into the cancer survivorship arena and the urgent need to do so. More specifically, all of the people living with cancer I was teaching as part of my cancer survivorship programmes were being treated with conventional medicine to great effect. But when these same people began to integrate Ayurveda safely and evidentially alongside their conventional care, something magical happened. They experienced a powerfully synergistic response in which the total benefit obtained was greater than the sum of the two individual approaches combined. In other words, when they started using Ayurvedic practices alongside their conventional cancer care, they obtained benefits that neither one of these modalities could provide on its own.

I saw first-hand the increased vibrancy, positivity and optimism with which they were living. I saw their fatigue melt away, their side effects diminish and in many cases their cancer markers, immune function and laboratory results improve. I even had the privilege, and continue to do so, of meeting many individuals who would themselves go on to become exceptional cancer patients.

It was during this time, when I was galvanised by the hugely positive benefits I was observing, and buoyed up by the relentless energy and positivity of my mentor, that my path forward became clear. To this day, I remember getting home late one night after delivering a cancer survivorship course to over forty women with breast and ovarian cancer, and, in a state of heightened clarity, writing a mission statement in my journal, which I still have all these years later. This is what I wrote:

> To empower the elevation and optimisation of human potential in the arenas of health, healing, longevity and the living of a purposeful life using the wisdom traditions of Ayurveda.

Over the last decade, this mission statement remains unchanged and every single day it continues to motivate and drive me. And fortunately, the validity of this mission statement in terms of the benefits of integrating evidence-based Ayurvedic practices into the arena of conventional medicine is gaining real and increasing traction. For example, at the time of writing, the National Health Service in the UK has funded clinical trials into the use of Ayurvedic herbs in general practice surgeries to reduce antibiotic prescribing, Nobel Prizes have been awarded to researchers studying circadian medicine concepts that align beautifully to Ayurvedic principles. Ayurvedic and Yogic practices now rank among the most commonly used techniques for supporting optimal mental and emotional health and some of the world's leading cancer hospitals, such as the Mayo Clinic and Memorial Sloan Kettering Cancer Center in the US, are studying and using Ayurveda and Ayurvedic herbs as part of their integrative cancer care packages.

That this is happening fills me with true optimism because, if the last fifteen years of work have taught me anything, they have taught me that when individuals living with cancer begin to effortlessly adopt and integrate the beautifully holistic practices of Ayurveda into their daily lives, their levels of health, vitality, wellbeing and optimism will soar. It very much appears that the world has awakened to the benefits of Ayurveda, and I truly hope and wish that this book will inspire you to harness these same benefits in your own life as you progress along your journey to thriving in the face of cancer.

## CHAPTER TWO

# Choosing Your Own Reality

*A child has no trouble in believing the unbelievable, nor does the genius or madman. It's only you and I, with our big brains and our tiny hearts, who doubt and overthink and hesitate.*

STEVEN PRESSFIELD, *Do the Work*

Upon finding out that you have cancer, your life changes overnight. A surge of emotions is unleashed into your consciousness: shock, anguish, regret and anger, to name just a few. In reality, all of these are masking a deeper primordial emotion: fear. This fear can come in myriad forms and take myriad expressions: fear of treatment, fear for our family, fear of loss and, at base, fear of death.

However, unlike the majority of the fears we encounter throughout our life, cancer is not an external threat that we can run from but a very internal one that is ever present. Many people with cancer talk of feeling betrayed by their own body and their own cells. This invariably leads to the asking of common questions such as: Why is this happening to me? Why now? How long do I have to live? Who will take care of my family? Am I going to die?

All of these questions, and the emotions that flow from them, are valid and normal when managing an illness such as cancer. And in and of themselves, they are not wrong or bad. However, they can quickly become damaging if we do not move beyond them into a new reality that we consciously create for ourselves and then live with a fierce intensity every single day. Doing so requires us to consciously and proactively delineate the illness and plot a multifaceted and integrated route back to wellness. This route begins with moving away from the more primordial, fear-based questions listed above to those that engender a more empowered and hope filled emotional space, such as:

What else can I do to improve my quality of life?
What more can I do to increase and improve my prognosis?
How can I stimulate my own natural healing mechanisms?
How can I maximise the impacts and benefits of the conventional treatments I am having?
How do I adopt a mindset of hope, optimism, autonomy and empowerment?
How can I empower myself to become an expert in navigating the field of cancer survivorship?
How do I, as a unique individual, become exceptional?

In short, how can I adopt, shape and hone a way of life that maximises both my health and my ability to thrive in the face of my diagnosis? With these questions asked and the empowered mindset they engender adopted, we take the first bold steps into what ultimately becomes a quantum leap into a field of possibility that has the potential to transform our health in unparalleled ways.

All of a sudden, the realm of impossible evaporates and in its place floods new options, new possibilities and new hope. And in many ways, this represents the very crux of this book: the realisation that when viewed through a different lens, the whole landscape typically associated with cancer looks vastly different. Through this lens, hopelessness becomes hopefulness. Helplessness becomes empowerment. Fearfulness becomes courageousness and ultimately, at the deepest level, impossible becomes possible. And amidst this dissolution, this breaking down of the old world order of cancer, a whole new realm of possibility emerges with regard to our ability to thrive in the face of cancer. And what I hope to show you in this book is how Ayurveda can be used as the lens through which this dissolution can be realised.

## 'Impossible Is Nothing' – A New Paradigm of Possibility

*Impossible is nothing.* The boxing fans out there will know that this famous statement was coined by Muhammad Ali, who in turn was paraphrasing Albert Einstein. What these two very different but equally virtuoso geniuses were both expressing was their absolute conviction that the only limiting factor in the sphere of possibility is the limitations imposed by our own thoughts and beliefs. In other words, if we think it possible, it becomes so. Nowhere is this belief more relevant, and indeed more important, than in the field of health and medicine. This is because so very often the beliefs that we maintain about any given disease, condition or statistic can act upon us in a way that makes that belief more likely to become reality. So common is this phenomenon that the field of health psychology has an actual label for it: a self-fulfilling prophecy. The more we believe in something, the more likely we are to act and behave, both consciously and subconsciously, in a way that will make that belief reach fruition.

And in many ways, this opens up a vital point in the study of exceptional cancer survival that I am sure most people will have heard of: the placebo response. A placebo response is defined as a positive, healing response that is produced in the body exclusively by our thoughts and expectations of a positive outcome. In contrast, and just as importantly, lies the counterbalance to the placebo called the nocebo response. This is defined as a negative and damaging physical response in the body that is produced exclusively by our fears and expectations.

The nocebo response is incredibly well documented within the clinical research, with studies showing that it can negatively impact upon health variables as diverse as chemotherapy-induced side effects and mood states, sleep quality and pain. As an example, a team of researchers recruited just under one hundred women and randomised them either to receive nocebo conditioning or to be in a control group. Those in the nocebo group watched a video of a model applying a completely benign ointment to her finger before acting out a severe pain response. The control group watched the same video but this time the model demonstrated no pain. When the same ointment (that contained no pain-inducing properties at all) was applied to the fingers of the control group, no pain was reported, which was to be expected. However, when the same ointment was applied to the fingers of those who had been manipulated via the nocebo response, a clinically significant level of pain was reported. Given the inert properties of the ointment, the only feasible explanation for this response was the power of participants' beliefs that they too would experience pain upon receipt of the ointment.

We are vulnerable to both the placebo and nocebo responses in all healthcare contexts, be that the receipt of antibiotics for a chest infection, receiving massage treatment from a therapist or undergoing talking therapies from a counsellor, to give but a few examples. But perhaps nowhere is the impact of the placebo and nocebo response more powerful and more profound than in the context of cancer. And perhaps the best documented example of just how profound this response can be lies in the incredible case of Mr Wright.[1]

## The Incredible Case of Mr Wright

While the exceptional healing responses initiated and experienced by Mr Wright are by no means unique or special, what makes them so important in our journey together through this book is that they were conducted and documented in an evidence-based setting with full clinical data and diagnostics to validate them. Therefore, they clearly document the potent seeds of exceptional that lie dormant in all of us, just waiting to germinate and bloom into full health.

Mr Wright had been diagnosed with an aggressive form of lymphoma (a type of cancer that develops in the cells of the lymphatic system) which had spread throughout much of his body. Bedridden and able to consume only liquids, he was given a few weeks to live and was admitted to a palliative care hospice in Long Beach, California. As Mr Wright wasted away and orange-sized tumours began appearing all over his body, he learned through a friend of a new cancer drug called Krebiozen, which was being shown to have miraculous results, particularly in those with advanced cancers.

Having discussed this new treatment option with his clinical care team, he begged his physician, Dr Philip West, to start treating him with Krebiozen. Despite some initial misgivings, Dr West agreed and his first injection was given late on Friday evening before Dr West finished work for the week. The following Monday, Dr West returned to his ward expecting to find his patient either dead or close to it. What he in fact found was something very different. Mr Wright wasn't dead. He didn't even appear to be ill. He was up out of his deathbed, walking around the ward, laughing and joking with the nurses and eating solid food for the first time in many months. His amazed doctors immediately ordered a raft of scans (subsequently reviewed and validated by an independent panel of doctors) to see exactly what was going on. These scans definitively revealed that his large, innumerable and incurable tumours had, in the words of Dr West, 'melted like snowballs on a hot stove'.

Several days later, and in even better health, the overjoyed Mr Wright was discharged and sent home, upon which he started playing golf and was by all accounts in tip-top health. But then, just over three months later, Mr Wright saw in the media that the miracle drug he was taking had been shown to be a quack therapy and was being removed as a recognised cancer treatment by the US Food and Drug Administration. Hearing this news was a huge emotional setback for Mr Wright. His joy, hope and optimism for a full recovery were dashed and he moved into a state of fear and hopelessness. He then suffered a near instant relapse, deteriorated quickly and within days was readmitted into hospital and back under the care of an even more baffled and confused Dr West.

What Dr West did next is now famous, or rather infamous, for his ethically justified decision to engage in a wholly unethical practice in the hope of helping his patient. This was a decision that nearly cost Dr West both his career and his reputation. Even more so, what the maverick Dr West did next produced one of the best-documented and clinically proven examples of the body's unique ability to induce truly staggering and in many ways unparalleled healing responses, even in those with the most advanced of cancers.

Dr West lied. More specifically, he went to great lengths to tell Mr Wright that the media reports about the failed efficacy of Krebiozen were untrue and misinformed. Furthermore, he explained calmly and sincerely that in all his years working as a doctor, Krebiozen really was the most miraculous cancer drug he has ever seen. He went as far as to say it may be the start of a final cure for cancer as we know it. Better still, he told Mr Wright that his clinic had been licensed to use a newly refined 'double strength' version of the drug, which had been shown to induce even more profound responses, particularly in those with the type of cancer Mr Wright was suffering from. He then injected this new double-strength Krebiozen into his patient. But what he in fact injected into Mr West wasn't double-strength Krebiozen at all. It was a completely inert placebo made with saline; just water and salt. Nothing active, nothing medicinal.

What happened next would change the way the healing mechanisms of the body are understood. Mr Wright got better. And not just a little better, but profoundly so. His orange-sized tumours melted away, he again rose from his deathbed and was again sent home. He lived in great health, with high levels of fitness and vitality for many months – until disaster struck. An unequivocal and definitive report was released showing that across all the research thus far conducted, Krebiozen was at best useless and at worst dangerous. Immediately hearing this, he contacted Dr West who was now no longer able to maintain the validity of his placebo and Mr Wright deteriorated rapidly. His tumours regrew, he was readmitted into hospice care for a third time and sadly died two days later.

The amazing example of Mr Wright, in equal parts tragic and empowering, provides a clear and telling example of just how powerful a role our beliefs and expectations can have upon the mechanisms, biology and growth of cancer. The truly amazing 'recovery-relapse' model that Mr Wright experienced had nothing to do with Krebiozen. It had been induced solely and exclusively by his mind and the power of his beliefs. Nothing more and nothing less. And because this case was conducted in a hospital setting with blood tests and scans to validate it, it proves beyond any questionable doubt that the beliefs we choose to cultivate have the ability to completely alter the trajectory of an illness. As to whether our mind has the ability to reliably achieve this is beyond doubt. The key question for all of us to ask is: 'How do we activate this mechanism in our own lives at will?'

As I shall discuss throughout this book, the ancient wisdom traditions of Ayurveda provide us with a profound framework for doing so in a way that is able to unlock the often-closed doors of healing. Unfortunately, however, it faces stern competition; the current medical paradigm, particularly in the sphere of oncology, makes this difficult to achieve as it is heavily vulnerable to the effects of negative beliefs. In the religion of academic medicine, statistics are the highest deity and are worshipped above all else. When the research states that stage 4 cancer is progressive and irreversible without exception, then for all people with stage 4 cancer that will be the outcome in every single case. Such a belief system prevails only in the absence of an alternative. Fortunately for us, it is as exciting as it is liberating that alternatives are coming thick and fast.

The growing and hugely exciting field of exceptional cancer survivorship research, such as that documented by Kelly A. Turner's bestselling book *Radical Remission* (which should be mandatory reading for all those living with cancer),[2] is unequivocally showing that it is a realistic possibility for those living with 'terminal' cancer – and therefore those living with less advanced cancers – to move into long-term cancer remission, regain full health and live a long and happy life, as we saw with Janet in the introduction. As such, it seems with absolute certainty that the flood gates are opening and a new paradigm is taking hold. This paradigm states that nothing is impossible because the research shows that everything is possible. People with terminal metastatic cancer have gone into complete remission. People with motor neurone disease have lived a long and full life. The human body has successfully destroyed the HIV virus. There is nothing to say that in the future, near or distant, a whole raft of progressive and irreversible diseases such as Parkinson's disease, Alzheimer's disease and generic stage 4 cancer won't be relabelled as reversible or, at the very least, containable.

And this is a view that sits right at the very heart of the Ayurvedic understanding of the treatment of disease and the cultivation of optimal health. Ayurveda acknowledges the view that if overall balance or homeostasis can be restored within the body, then so too can health. In fact, this concept of the restoration of balance is, when all is said and done, the whole and exclusive aim of Ayurveda. Why, when living an Ayurvedic lifestyle, do we adopt simple and sustainable dietary and lifestyle modifications, such as including all of the six tastes in our daily meals, waking and going to bed at the correct times, practising yoga and meditation, and integrating herbal medicines into our daily regime? (We will be exploring and unpicking these topics in subsequent chapters.) All these specific examples have clinically proven impacts upon the physiological workings of the body that can be observed and documented via Western clinical assessments such as blood tests and hormone profiling. But above and beyond this, these types of Ayurvedic modalities are adopted into our lives, at base, to keep our *doshas*, or bodily constitutions, in balance. In this way, we ensure that all our cells, organs, hormones, immune variables, biochemistry, emotions, beliefs and attitudes are operating from a place of profound balance. And with that will always come an elevation in health, wellbeing and longevity.

So, what I hope to show you in this book is not just *what* is possible with regard to optimising the healing capacity of the body, but more importantly *how* to achieve this. And to do that, we firstly have to open the door on what for me is without question the most exciting and paradigm-changing model of holistic, whole-person medicine in the world: Ayurveda.

## Ayurveda: The Science of Optimal Living

While I have been fortunate to have been immersed in Ayurveda from a very early age, when I first began to study and research it clinically, I felt like all the questions I had been asking around the cultivation of optimal health had been answered and that I had entered the promised land of healing.

Originating in India over five thousand years ago, Ayurveda represents an ancient science of healing based on a deep understanding of the inherent truths of the human body and mind. More specifically, Ayurveda provides us with a time-tested blueprint for harnessing these truths in the quest for the cultivation of optimal health and the effective and holistic treatment of illness and disease. Central and fundamental to the entire clinical application of Ayurveda are the three doshas: *vata*, *pitta* and *kapha*. These doshas represent our unique mind-body constitution, the very foundation of what makes me 'me' and you 'you' at the physical, psychological and emotional level.

If you are new to the world of Ayurveda, it can initially be helpful to view the doshas as a broader and most holistic form of genetics. In this way, the colour of your eyes, the quality of your hair, the robustness of your immunity, your psychological likes and dislikes, how your digestive system works, your sleeping patterns and every other subtle nuance of the completely unique and amazing individual that is you is based upon your doshic balance.

Every individual has all three doshas working within them, but it is the unique ratio of these three doshas in any given individual that is directly responsible for the make-up of that person's individual mind-body constitution, or, in Western parlance, their genetic profile. Ayurveda says that we are each born with a completely unique doshic ratio called *prakruti*, which equates to our individual genetic blueprint – our identity. This will always remain within us and is unchangeable, in the same way that the colour of our eyes and the shape of our tongue are. Our prakruti represents our best possible physiological and emotional state and is responsible for the cultivation of our highest levels of health, happiness and longevity.

However, we also have a more variable and negatively construed doshic balance called our *vikruti*, which literally translates from the Sanskrit as 'to deviate away from our nature'. In other words, if prakruti represents our optimal state of physiological, psychological and emotional balance –and where we unleash our most powerful healing mechanisms – vikruti represents a move away from this. Vikruti is the 'here and now' ratio of the three doshas and is the net result of all the influences around us, such as weather, food, work, family and stress.

For example, if you were to rush home from work late one evening, miss dinner and in a state of overwhelm and stress stay up working on a business project until the early hours of the morning, a little bit of vikruti will be added to your body and mind, moving you a little further away from your optimal, health-promoting prakruti. If this happens day after day, more and more vikruti will be progressively added as the stress, overwork and broken sleep accumulate. If this continues for any meaningful period of time, vikruti will eventually accumulate to a point in which it will break through into a symptomatic state: overt anxiety, fatigue, tension headaches, stress, acid reflux or myriad other presentations.

The best way of understanding these two types of doshic balances is to view prakruti as the hard wooden surface of a beautiful and strong mahogany table; it is solid and stable and doesn't move or change. This represents our very highest level of health and vitality. Vikruti is like a layer of dust on the surface of this table that is constantly changing in the face of innumerable influences impacting upon us. This dust represents the seeds of physical damage, trauma and disease, which, left unchecked, will ultimately lead to a fully fledged health crisis. Ayurveda says it is our aim to remove this layer of dust and through doing so return to our original and optimal constitutional balance (prakruti), which is the foundation of optimal health and healing. When it comes to the Ayurvedic management of cancer, removing or clearing this vikruti is vital. This is because it is the build-up of vikruti over many years that leads to the pathological changes in our cells that are ultimately responsible for the development of malignancy in the first place. All of the practices, approaches and interventions discussed in this book are designed to help remove vikruti, the dust, from the hard clean surface of prakruti, and through doing so awaken the body's inherent ability to restore health.

It is also vital to note that the dust of vikruti can settle in our mind as well as our physical body. In many ways, the exceptional healing responses that were observed in Mr Wright were brought about by the removal of the mental vikruti of fear, hopelessness and helplessness that allowed the full blossoming of the hope, optimism and belief that underpinned his miraculous journey. Thus, while many of the approaches we shall be discussing over the coming chapters have a very physical orientation, particularly with regard to the activation of the myriad evidence-based anti-cancer mechanisms operating within the body, it is just as important that we also address mental and emotional vikruti too.

The recommendations we will be exploring are suitable for everyone, irrespective of their doshic balance. However, in certain instances the success of these interventions can be greatly enhanced by knowing the state of your unique vikruti right now. Knowing this will allow you to tailor the advice provided in a much more individualised way. For instance, if your vikruti is very vata dominant, it is important that you emphasise a higher intake of certain foods, herbs and spices than if your vikruti was very pitta dominant. Similarly, if you are experiencing digestive symptoms such as bloating and wind (very vata-based symptoms), this would require different recommendations than if you were experiencing digestive symptoms such as acid reflux (a very pitta-based symptom). Spending some time working out your unique vikruti can be tremendously helpful at this point in our journey together. To facilitate this, I have included a Vikruti Assessment Questionnaire for you to complete in appendix 1, which will allow you to accurately do so. Similarly, in appendix 1 you will also find a weblink to my free Introduction to the Doshas course. This provides a deep immersion in and exploration of the doshas for the interested reader who is looking to learn more about this fascinating topic.

## The Ayurvedic View and Understanding of Cancer

Ayurveda is the guardian of over five thousand years of knowledge regarding the promotion of perfect health, the optimisation of human longevity and the treatment of illness and disease. Included within this knowledge is an incredibly holistic and beautifully empowering view and understanding of cancer management. I believe that this view has a huge amount to offer those living with cancer in the West. And so, before we progress onto the next chapter, it is essential for us to explore this beautifully holistic and uniquely insightful way in which Ayurveda understands the process of both cancer formation and, more importantly, cancer destruction. To begin this unique exploration, we firstly have to ask ourselves an intriguing question:

Are all the cells within our body, both healthy and cancerous, capable of thinking and expressing emotions?

This is a question that we have to lead with because in many ways it lays the physiological foundation of how we begin to unpick and unlock the move into exceptional. The proven answer to this question, as strange as it sounds, is that yes – every cell in our body is capable of experiencing and expressing emotions. And this fact is vital to our understanding of how cancer works. Moreover, it reminds us of why the holistic understanding of cancer that Ayurveda advocates is so important and so relevant in the cutting-edge world of twenty-first-century medicine.

To begin to understand how all the cells in our body, and not just our brain cells, are capable of thinking and expressing emotions in this way, we have to move back in time to the 1970s when a brilliant young scientist called Candace Pert published clinical research that caused a collective gasp from around the scientific world. For what Dr Pert had discovered was the now famous neuropeptides, more commonly known as our 'molecules of emotion'.[3] These molecules of emotion explain how every thought, emotion, belief, hope and attitude we experience in our mind goes on to be directly mirrored and experienced by the cells in our physical body. And this emotional mirroring imparts a truly profound and perhaps unrivalled impact – for better or for worse – upon the health of those cells, depending upon the quality of the thoughts being expressed. She had discovered, for the very first time, a scientifically proven model of mind-over-matter at the cellular level.

Of central importance to those living with cancer, what Dr Pert had uniquely and specifically discovered, was that each and every one of the millions of cells that make up our immune system have neuropeptide receptors on them. Neuropeptide receptors are a type of neuroreceptor (also called a neurotransmitter receptor) that specifically binds with neuropeptides. At the foundational level, neuroreceptors are ultimately what allow our body to talk to itself. More specifically, neuroreceptors allow one cell to directly communicate a message to another cell in a distant part of the body. In many ways, it is helpful to visualise this as two different types of cells, operating in different and distant parts of the body, holding a walkie-talkie tuned to the same radio frequency. By being connected to this frequency, the cells are able to talk to each other in a bidirectional manner to convey vital information relevant to the optimal functioning of the body, the preservation of health and the suppression of disease.

The crucial point that Dr Pert identified, particularly in the context of cancer management, was that our immune cells possess these neuropeptide receptors. What this meant was that the millions of immune cells that are constantly patrolling our body in a never-ending quest to prevent and contain cancer (and other pathogens) were in constant, reactive and direct communication with the nervous system at every second of every minute of the day. But here comes the crux: our nervous system includes the brain, which in turn contains our thoughts and emotions. So, in a practical sense, the discovery of neuropeptide receptors on our immune cells means that every thought, emotion, belief, attitude, hope, dream and expectation we experience is communicated to, and goes on to directly and quantifiably impact upon, the workings of every cell in the vastness of our immune system. In other words, our emotions are constantly 'talking' to our immune cells. And crucially, it is the content of this dialogue that goes on to directly impact upon the functioning of our immune cells, for better or for worse.

For example, if we are consumed by fear, anxiety, hopelessness, helplessness, disempowerment, stress and any other negative emotional state, these very same emotions are, at the molecular level, experienced and expressed by our immune cells. And what happens when our immune cells express stress, anxiety and fear? They work less efficiently and less effectively. Their intelligence falters, their impact weakens, their reactivity slows. This now explains how and why stress, as a singular example, is clinically proven to suppress immune activity and increase our risk factors for infections and cancer cell proliferation. To put this into a practical context, it also explains a landmark study from the US that revealed that over 70 per cent of those diagnosed with cancer had experienced a significant life stressor in the twelve to sixteen months prior to diagnosis.[4] The theory now being that this significant life stressor negatively impacted upon the thoughts, emotions and attitudes of those experiencing it. These emotions were then similarly expressed by the immune cells, resulting in significant immune suppression that may have allowed a cancerous cell mutation to go unnoticed for long enough for a symptomatic tumour to form.

Fortunately, however, the opposite is also true. When we consciously cultivate a mindset and belief system that radiates hope, optimism, empowerment, vitality, health, recovery, survival, love, the realisation of dreams and any other positive emotional state, these same emotions are in turn experienced and expressed by our immune cells. And how do immune cells bathed in this kind of emotional vitality behave? They become strong, numerous, hyper-intelligent, active, powerful and domineering. In other words, exactly the kind of immune system we need when facing the threat of cancer.

Could this mechanism explain the amazing case of Mr Wright we discussed earlier? When presented with the completely unexpected opportunity of hope in what was otherwise a hopeless situation, did the emotions that stemmed from this – optimism, gratitude, excitement, amazement, empowerment, control – directly invigorate his immune system in such a way as to bring about the complete dissolution of his extensive cancer burden? Was it this that allowed his multiple tumours to, in his doctor's words, melt 'like snowballs on a hot stove'? To date, this seems like the most plausible and evidence-based mechanism underpinning exceptional cancer recoveries. That is not to say that it is the only mechanism at play, but it is almost certainly a vital one. And the reason this is so important is because it provides a beautifully holistic bridge that joins the Western understanding of exceptional cancer recovery with its Ayurvedic counterpart.

In the Ayurvedic understanding of cancer, every cell in the body is an individual centre of awareness and consciousness that is capable of experiencing and expressing emotions, just as we have seen in the work of Dr Candace Pert. As humans, we are prized as perhaps being the only species in the world that is conscious of its consciousness. But that consciousness, the consciousness that is allowing you to hold, read and interpret this book, is not made solely by the brain. It is ultimately the result of the sum of all the individual centres of consciousness of the trillions of cells that make up your body. In Ayurveda, this cellular consciousness is called *ahamkara*, which conceptually translates as the 'I maker'.

At the broader level, ahamkara is what keeps the world in order and prevents, for example, an apple tree from producing a cucumber. As silly as that sounds, it is an important point. Every apple seed that has ever existed contained within it the ahamkara that says, 'I am an apple.' Through doing so, this ensures the correct form, structure and functioning of the seed in such a way as to make new apples and, therefore, new apple trees to preserve the balanced order of the natural world.

So, too, in our species. Think right back to your conception. The moment you were conceived, when ovum and sperm met, it was the ahamkara in these two cells that informed and regulated the progressive and continual division of new cells until, nine months later, the beautiful and completely unique human that is you was born. And once you were born, it was the ahamkara inherent in each of the fifty trillion cells in your body that ensured the collective and harmonious functioning of your entire physiology. It is the ahamkara acting in your liver cells that ensures these cells work and behave as liver cells and not eye cells. It is the ahamkara of your kidney cells that allows them to purify the water in our body, the ahamkara of your brain cells that allows you to possess rational thought and the ahamkara of your optic nerves that allows you to see, experience and enjoy the beauty of the natural world all around us.

Thus, in essence, it is the ahamkara operating individually in each and every cell of the body that maintains the collective and unified health of the body in such a way as to prevent imbalance and disease from establishing. So, what happens to allow a normal, healthy cell to mutate into a damaged cancerous one? Ultimately the ahamkara of that first initial cancerous cell (and by inference all subsequent cancerous cells) becomes confused, isolated, lost and unable to communicate effectively with all the other healthy cells in the body. It fails to understand its role and purpose. It has lost its sense of self. This confusion in the cellular consciousness can be caused by many variables: carcinogenic compounds, loneliness, poor nutrition, toxins, stress and genetics, to name just a few.

Once a cell loses its ahamkara, catastrophic changes begin to occur. In the Ayurvedic tradition, such a cell becomes completely isolated from all the other healthy cells in the body. The functioning of such a cell becomes unrecognisable when viewed in comparison to a healthy cell; its cellular, metabolic and biochemical actions bear no resemblance to that of a healthy cell. Sensing its lost unity with its healthy cellular neighbours, the cancerous cell begins acting as a lone ranger. Realising that it no longer benefits from the self-regulating and self-protecting mechanisms of the body in the way healthy cells do, it begins to fear for its survival. It no longer 'feels' part of the body but rather an isolated renegade operating within it. Thus, from the Ayurvedic perspective, the cancer cell inherently recognises that the body will no longer act to protect it and has only one option left available to it if it is to secure its own survival: self-replication.

It is at this point that the journey of cancer begins. The entire ahamkara of the now cancerous cell changes from a selfless focus on optimising the health of the body to a mindless and self-absorbed obsession with self-preservation. As that first malignant cell divides into two, a new cancerous cell with the same damaged sense of ahamkara is created. This in turn divides and divides again as cancer cell proliferation gathers pace until a large enough cancer burden is created to become symptomatic and subsequently diagnosed. This is the vikruti, the dust on the solid table of prakruti, to which we previously referred.

On the one hand, we can see clear, immutable synergy with the Western neuropeptide research of Dr Candace Pert: cells, both healthy and unhealthy, being able to experience and express emotions, which in turn go on to inform the very ways those cells behave. On the other hand, what this uniquely Ayurvedic view of cancer provides us with is a beautifully holistic framework for its holistic management. This framework requires of us to progress down two avenues of management at the same time. The first avenue focuses on the adoption of evidence-based cancer survivorship practices that have been shown to help suppress the activity and growth of cancer cells. To achieve this, the full arsenal of Ayurvedic treatments (alongside its conventional counterparts) is pressed into service: anti-cancer nutritional approaches, herbal medicines, lifestyle practices and much else besides.

But another equally, and perhaps more profound, avenue of treatment is also employed. This avenue focuses on the view that the surest way of encouraging the body to rid itself of cancer is to actually intellectualise the cancer cells in such a way as to make them feel safe, secure and part of the collective body once again. As their consciousness elevates, as their original, health-preserving ahamkara returns and as their molecules of emotion become more positive, they let go of their death grip on self-preservation.

If we approach this singularly Ayurvedic understanding of cancer through the lens of Western clinical research, we can see this concept playing out in all its wonderful holism. As a single example among many, consider why it is that a seemingly irrelevant practice such as meditation has been proven to induce a process called apoptosis, or programmed cell death, in cancer cells. There appears to be no obvious link between how and why the silent repetition of a mantra should be able to directly signal to a rogue, confused and lost cancer cell to passively lay down its arms and die. Could it be that through the deeply consciousness-elevating impacts of meditation, the original and previously lost ahamkara of the cancer cell is returned? And through its return, the focus of the cancer cell moves from one of fear and self-preservation to one that instead prioritises the overall health of its host, the body? And could not this reawakening then motivate the cancer cell to end its cellular rebellion, lay down arms and die?

Similar examples exist for myriad other lifestyle practices, such as yoga, gratitude techniques, vision boarding and visualisation. All of these important approaches elevate our consciousness to new heights, and they do likewise for all the cells in the body, including cancerous ones. And this elevation in consciousness has no choice but to reawaken the original, health-preserving ahamkara that existed in each cancer cell before it became rogue. Thus, in helping to guide and support those with cancer, Ayurveda advocates that we walk each of these two avenues at the same time in the belief that they both lead onto the path of exceptional. The aim of the following chapters is to signpost the way.

# CHAPTER THREE

# The Biology of Hope
*Unlocking the Gates of Exceptional*

> *I have become my own version of an optimist. If I can't make it through one door, I'll go through another door – or I'll make a door. Something terrific will come no matter how dark the present.*
>
> RABINDRANATH TAGORE

As we begin our journey into the realm of exceptional cancer survivorship, it is imperative that our very first stop alights at the luminous gates of the human mind and all the limitless potential for healing that is to be found there. In subsequent chapters, we will journey into areas of healing that we more commonly associate with cancer survivorship, such as diet and nutrition, immune support, herbal medicines, gut health and much else besides. But the successful implementation of such practices is itself dependent upon one thing: our ability to unleash the power of the human mind and bring this to bear on the reality of cancer in such a way as to transform that reality. The implications of this upon the activation of the healing mechanisms of the body are profound for the simple fact that the first step in reaching for exceptional is cultivating the belief that it is possible. Not simply a transient 'fingers crossed and hope for the best' belief that is easily railroaded by discouraging statistics or setbacks, but rather an all-consuming belief in the possibility of survival that infuses every atom of our being.

Working to cultivate this kind of belief system is a transformative process. Our levels of emotional vitality soar as psychological states such as hope, optimism, positivity, excitement and control become our default outlook in day-to-day life. Similarly, and as we shall explore in detail as this chapter unfolds, cultivating this kind of belief system can also radically alter the neurobiology of the body in a way that promotes enhanced physiological healing. A multidisciplinary foundation of scientific evidence now shows that the exceptional healing mechanisms of the body that lie inherent in every one of us are best and most fully mobilised when the mind says 'yes'.[1] In other words, we have to create a new reality around our health and survival that we genuinely believe is possible for us to realise, irrespective of the statistics we are facing. If we can do this, we can do anything.

The aim of this chapter, and the next, is to explore how practices such as goal setting, guided imagery and meditation can be used to cultivate this restructuring and reordering of our belief systems in a way that can so powerfully impact upon a whole host of survival mediated mechanisms, right down to facilitating increased survival times in those with advanced cancer.[2]

This fundamental role of the mind in the activation of healing is a concept that holds centre stage in the arena of Ayurveda, which states that the health and functionality of the entire body – our DNA, chromosomes, cells, tissues and organs – is at the foundational level the net result of our level of consciousness. When we are able to transcend our rational, reactive mind in a way that moves it beyond the labels of ill health, ageing and disease, we are instead able to move into a completely free and liberated state of consciousness called *mukta*. The cultivation of mukta is vital in our quest for optimal health as it is responsible for establishing that profound state of balance – homeostasis in Western parlance and prakruti in Ayurveda – which is the foundational physiological state from which healing occurs.

Unfortunately, however, dealing with and managing cancer is an inherently unbalancing process that can, if not properly managed, create a negative feedback loop; increasing fear, anxiety and uncertainty directly suppresses a host of crucial physiological mechanisms relevant to cancer survivorship, such as immune activity, gut health, sleep quality and inflammatory mechanisms.[3] This suppression, in turn, robs us of our highest levels of physical vitality, strength and healing capacities when we need them the most. It is vital that we find a way out of this vicious circle. And the way out requires us to look within. Specifically, it requires us to harness the infinitely creative power of our mind and use this to recreate our current reality from one that is predominantly disease focused to one that is predominantly health focused.

It is the creation of this new type of reality that is synonymous with the cultivation of an unwavering, unquestionable and unequivocal belief in our ability to go on to regain our most vital levels of health, even in the face of a cancer diagnosis. Change at this level of consciousness will always be the most profound because it is the only change that can, in and of itself, go on to permeate every single part of our body and mind. In many ways, this recreation of our reality and the shift in consciousness that it engenders is one of the most powerful ways of removing the 'dust' of vikruti from the hard wooden table of prakruti that we discussed in the previous chapter.

So, as we begin our discussion of this transformative model of healing, the very first thing we need to explore is the sheer subjectivity of what we call reality. Traditionally, when we think of reality, we think of something that is immutably real, objective and the same for everyone. That beautiful red rose that you can see in your garden is clearly and definitively red. A frosty winter morning is singularly and quantifiably cold for everyone. The brick wall in your living room is obviously and unquestionably solid. All these examples, and virtually every other facet of daily life, are objective realities that are the same for everyone experiencing them. Such a statement looks and sounds to be true until we change the lens through which we perceive them. For example:

- The beautiful red rose in your garden that is so objectively red actually isn't. Observed through the eyes and nervous system of your dog or cat, or someone living with colour blindness, it wouldn't appear red at all but rather a muddy brown colour. What colour is it then – red or brown? Who is correct – us or the dog?
- Take again that frosty winter morning. If you live on the south coast of England where I live, frost is a rarity. Thus, a thick frost would be perceived by the morning weather forecasters and the people living here as being exceptionally and unequivocally 'cold'. But for an Inuit living deep within the Arctic Circle who is used to surviving in winter temperatures as low as −40°C, the frosty morning in southern England that I call cold would be positively balmy. Who is correct? Is it cold or balmy?
- We can go even further with this recreation of reality. Take something that is physically and immutably real: a brick wall. A brick wall is unquestionably solid and impossible to pass through. That's the reality of a brick wall. Or is it? That reality only applies to objects with a certain atomic size; humans can't walk through walls because we are too big to pass through the atomic structure making up the wall. But sound waves

and X-rays, for example, can pass through because they are small enough to slip through the atoms and molecules making up the wall. Therefore, is a brick wall solid and unpassable or not? It depends.

The list goes on, but the point remains: nothing that exists in the field of human consciousness is a definitive reality. Nothing at all. And this subjective interpretation of the nature of reality is of fundamental importance in relation to healing because the questioning and recreation of our reality applies as much to clinical variables and clinical outcomes as it does to brick walls, roses and weather conditions. In other words, when it comes to clinical status, there is no objective reality.

Chemotherapeutic treatment is a fantastic example here. The common side effects that so often occur in those being treated with chemotherapy are incredibly well documented, such as nausea and vomiting. And yet, compelling evidence shows that it is not just the drug itself that causes these side effects but also the reality we create around the drug in our own minds. Consider the findings from a fascinating study conducted at the Wilmot Cancer Institute (previously the University of Rochester Cancer Center) in the US.[4] This study demonstrated that close to 50 per cent of people due to start chemotherapy for the first time actually experienced the primary symptoms of treatment *before* the treatment began. Why? The analysis showed it was because they believed they would experience these side effects as an inevitable response to their treatment because their oncologist told them so. But – and this is a really important but – an alternative positive recreation of this reality was also possible. Specifically, and somewhat amazingly, none of the patients who believed they would not experience nausea and vomiting went on to experience such symptoms. Not one. This is an incredibly powerful example of the physiological reshaping of clinical reality exclusively by our minds and our expectations.

But the crux of this issue – and the reason why it is of such tremendous importance with regard to healing – is that the interpretation of reality occurs wholly and exclusively within our mind and nervous system. Neurologically speaking, it is now generally accepted that the only thing a human being can ever experience is their own nervous system.[5] And the nervous system includes the objective brain and the subjective mind, both of which are always under our conscious control.

It can often feel like this is not the case but, psychologically speaking, it is a foundational truth. For example, if someone were to aggressively cut in front of me when I was driving home after a stressful day at work, my immediate response might be anger and frustration. This may feel like a reaction I am powerless to control but it actually isn't. I could choose to not respond that way. I could choose to acknowledge that perhaps the person driving that car has a sick child at home and they are rushing back to help. This brings empathy into the equation and with it the decision to react not aggressively but rather with kindness. It cultivates the empowerment of choice over the impotency of reaction. In many ways, this concept is best articulated by the literary genius of William Shakespeare when Hamlet laments that 'there is nothing either good or bad, but thinking makes it so'. This striking observation is of fundamental importance as it highlights the all-powerful role played by the thinker (that is to say, you and I) in the creation of our reality – be that the treatment side effects we experience, our response to traffic, our belief in our ability to become exceptional or virtually any other experience we encounter in each moment of our lives.

If we then take this line of enquiry a step further, we can see that if the interpretation of reality occurs exclusively in our mind (which it does), and if we have autonomous control over our mind (which we unequivocally do), then by default we are also blessed to have complete control over how we shape reality; it is ours to do what we want with. There are many famous examples of the power of this kind of interpretation playing out in some of the worst cases of human baseness. Viktor Frankl transforming the reality of the Nazi concentration camps during World War II via the practice of extreme gratitude. Nelson Mandela transforming the reality of his thirty-year incarceration on Robben Island into a profound opportunity for learning and self-development that led to the freeing of a nation. Stephen Hawking transforming the imprisoned and dependent state of his physical illness into the boundless intellectual exploration of the infinity of the cosmos. These are towering examples of how we can bend the reality of the world we inhabit and the situations we face by nothing more than an empowered shift in consciousness.

What these seismic shifts in consciousness highlight is that, irrespective of the situations we are facing, we can harness the immense power of our mind to completely alter and restructure the nature of the reality we currently inhabit. The deprivation, hardships and hunger that Viktor Frankl experienced in the concentration camps were the same as everyone else living alongside him. And yet through a shift in consciousness, he was able to positively alter the nature of that reality and in doing so stay strong in mind and body. And, crucially for us, Western scientific evidence now shows that this consciousness-created shift in reality can induce a corresponding alteration in the physiology of the body in a way that matches the new reality we have created for ourselves; believe healing and recovery is possible, and create enough accuracy around this reality, and the body will move in such a way as to maximise the ability of that reality to reach fruition.

As an illuminating example of this process, consider this now famous study exploring the role of the mind upon surgical healing.[6] Individuals with painful osteoarthritis in their knee joint were randomly assigned to have either: 1) surgery to scrape damaged cartilage from within the knee joint; 2) surgery to wash out the knee joint with saline to remove the inflammation-causing debris; or 3) 'sham surgery' in which the patient's knee would be opened up and then sewn back together with no surgical intervention. All patients received the same preoperative procedures, all were wheeled into surgery and all were fully anaesthetised. The results were fascinating. *All* the patients reported clinically significant improvements in knee pain and mobility, including those who had had the pretend surgery – they demonstrated the same level of clinical success and improvement as those who had had the real surgery. Crucially, when followed up, these gains were still present six months and six years later. These are profound findings. And the only mechanism that can explain these kinds of results is that a shift in their reality – 'I am having surgery and thus will feel better' – was responsible for the clinical success observed. But before we explore the application of such actions in our own lives in relation to cancer survivorship, it will be helpful for us to detour to a cold, wet running track in Oxford in 1954, when Roger Bannister broke the four-minute mile. Here we see a fantastically clear example of just how powerful an impact a reinterpretation of reality can have upon altering and unleashing the full physiological workings of the body in a way that opens up the doors of impossible.

## What Roger Bannister Can Teach Us About Exceptional Cancer Survivorship

In many ways, Roger Bannister's quest to become the first person to break the four-minute mile exemplifies the qualities that are required by those living with cancer in their pursuit of exceptional survival: conviction, inner belief, optimism and a refusal to buy into the negativity of those who question their conviction. And while Roger Bannister's application of becoming exceptional occurs within the sporting arena, it has subsequently gone on to become a clarion call for all those challenging the status quo in a diverse array of fields including the worlds of business, health, science, leadership and human rights. And as we shall now see, it provides us with such an incredible insight into why the cultivation of the correct mindset and belief system represents the necessary foundation from which all exceptional healing is subsequently built upon.

On 6 May 1954, Roger Bannister made sporting history by becoming the first person to break the four-minute mile with a time of three minutes, fifty-nine and four-tenths of a second. In the annals of history and world records, the story ends there. But behind this headline is an even more incredible story and for us a more important one. And that story is that elite athletes had been seriously chasing the goal of breaking the four-minute mile in a systematic way since 1886. As the decades went by, it became the athletic equivalent of the space race. Athletes from all around the world were competing to become the first person to break this elusive Everest of athletic achievement as testament to the supremacy of their nation. And yet no one could do it. The best athletes with the best coaches in the best environmental conditions were simply unable to get even close to breaking the four-minute barrier. By the early 1950s, there was a growing consensus from the athletes, coaches and sports scientists that it was looking increasingly likely that it might be physiologically and bio-mechanically impossible for a human being to cover a mile in less than four minutes. It had nothing to do with fitness, training, technique or conditions. It was simply that asking a man to cover that distance in that time was akin to asking him to walk on water: both were physiological impossibilities. In so many ways, this mirrors the challenges that are often faced by those living with advanced cancer in their quest to becoming exceptional. Someone is diagnosed with a stage 4 cancer and the prognosis is that the cancer is incurable and aggressive, and the only treatment options available are palliative rather than curative. All hope is removed and long-term survival becomes impossible in exactly the same way that breaking the four-minute mile was viewed as being impossible. However, a simple shift in reality can unlock the doors of impossible and free the possible lurking within. And, in the context of breaking the elusive four-minute mile, it was Roger Bannister who held the key.

At the time, Bannister was an amateur runner and full-time student with no coach, no support and no professional training. When he announced his intention to break the four-minute mile using his own private training and preparation methods, he was ridiculed and dismissed as a disillusioned and idealistic amateur looking for his five minutes of fame. Until one cold, wet morning at a small athletics meet in Oxford when Bannister laced on his shoes, took to the track and achieved the impossible.

But it is what happened next that is so relevant to the arena of cancer survivorship. Remember that since 1886 hundreds and hundreds of athletes from around the world had been striving to break the four-minute mile without success. From 1946 to 1954, the intensity reached fever pitch and it was an athletic obsession for dozens of countries and their top athletes to break through this unbreakable barrier. No one could do it; it was impossible. But herein lies the crux: once Roger Bannister did it, so too did *everyone else*! Less than a month after Bannister entered the history books, the Australian runner John Landy not only broke the four-minute mile but shaved an unimaginable second off the time. Then, three runners broke the four-minute mile in *a single race*.

Over the following two years, almost all of the world's top runners who had tried unsuccessfully for years to achieve this feat achieved their goal. How and why was this possible? What had changed that allowed the accepted impossibility of the task to morph into possible literally overnight? None of the key variables relevant to elite athletic performance – the athlete's fitness, coaching, age, weight, nutrition or equipment – had changed. In fact, every facet of what is required to successfully break the four-minute mile remained the same post Roger Bannister except one: the knowledge that it was possible. And with that knowledge, everything changed. The walls of doubt fell and the concept of the task being impossible dissolved like the mirage it always was. The runners of the past had been held back exclusively by the mindset that it was impossible. In their mind, it couldn't be done and so it wasn't; their body said no because their mind said no. But as soon as it was done, the self-limiting doubt was removed. And its removal then unleashed a latent power in the physiology of the athletes that allowed them to run in a way that they couldn't run before. In short, the knowledge that something was possible was the very mechanism that allowed it to become so. This relationship is in many ways best portrayed pictorially, as shown in figure 3.1.

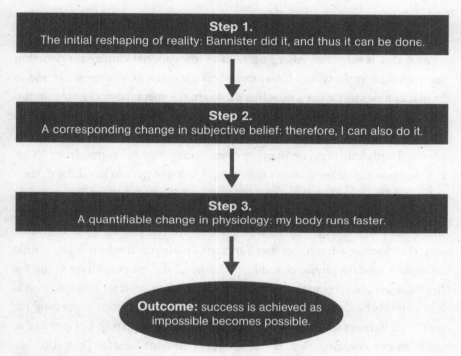

Figure 3.1. The reshaping of reality can change the outcome.

It is almost impossible to over-emphasise the importance of this example in relation to exceptional cancer survivorship. We have to believe fully and unequivocally, at the conscious and subconscious level, in our ability to regain full vital health and in our ability to enjoy many more decades of bright, vibrant life. Irrespective of the clinical situation you are facing, the beacon of hope that long-term survival is within reach must always burn brightly. We must harness the exploding foundation of clinical evidence that testifies to our unquestionable ability to become exceptional in the face of impossible odds and use this to fuel a level of hope and trust in our ability to regain health that acknowledges no limits. This is not a move into denial – far from it. Rather, this is about absolutely and always fully acknowledging our diagnosis: this is crucial. But it is also about the vehement refusal to do likewise for our prognosis. Prognoses are built upon historical data that have no direct bearing upon you as a precious and completely unique individual. In this context, the advice attributed to Albert Einstein can be tremendously helpful: 'We cannot solve our problems with the same thinking we used when we created them.' So, too, with us. To solve the problem of cancer in our own individual lives, we need to move our mind to a place that is beyond it.

And this is why the emerging field of exceptional cancer survivorship research is so important: it blows the lid off the concept of impossible and in its place shows just what's possible; these are the metaphorical four-minute-mile-breakers of the cancer survivorship world. Nowadays, it is difficult to find an example of a terminal stage 4 cancer that someone hasn't successfully survived with long term or, in many cases, completely recovered from.[7] This is a vital point because it shows that even if just one person has done it, then theoretically so can another. This is our Roger Bannister moment: knowing it can be done and achieving it. Knowing someone else has done it and using that knowledge to fuel our own belief that we too can do it. In the same way that knowing Bannister had successfully broken the four-minute mile unleashed a latent physiological response in all the other athletes vying for the same goal, so it is with the body's latent healing powers. The question is less 'can this be done?' and more 'what is stopping this from happening for me?' The barriers and enablers in this context exist squarely, but not exclusively, in our consciousness as our thoughts and our beliefs. Therefore, we can take the model used to illustrate the Roger Bannister effect and apply it specifically to cancer survivorship, as shown in figure 3.2.

The now conventionally accepted and acknowledged role of the human mind as a governor and regulator of healing is transforming the way medicine is viewed and understood. What this research shows is that the body is fluid and changeable and that if something is broken, it can be fixed. Ayurveda uses a beautiful analogy to portray this state of flux: 'you cannot step into the same river twice.' We see this as an absolute truth. When you step out of a river and then step back in again, you are not standing in the same river as before. Rather, you would be standing in completely new water, and thus in a completely new river. So, too, with the body; it is continually changing, modifying and altering. The body you inhabit today is not the body you will inhabit tomorrow at the atomic and cellular level. Evidence shows that over any twelve-month period, 98 per cent of the atomic make-up of your body is replaced. This is bodily renewal at the most profound level.

Our challenge is to ensure that this process of renewal is being used to cultivate health rather than promote disease. And to do that, we need to enter a place where cancer no longer exists, a place in fact where it is impossible for

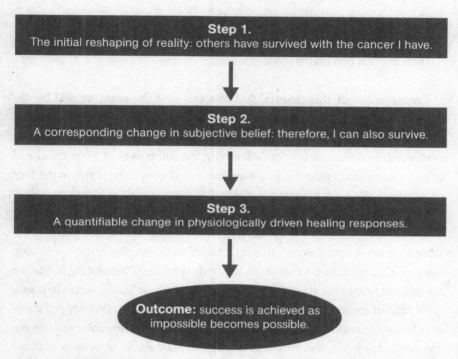

Figure 3.2. Reshaping reality can change our body's healing responses.

cancer to ever exist. This is a place that is beyond illness, beyond disease and, in the purest sense, beyond death. That place is our consciousness or true Self. For when we access that place, we harness healing mechanisms that are for most people most of the time completely untapped. And, as we have been exploring all the way through this chapter, that mechanism is the mind.

But like any great tool, it is only powerful in the hands of a master who knows how to use it. So it is with the mind. We have to learn how to access its latent power in the pursuit of healing and then know how to unleash it in an effective and replicable way. Doing so requires us to firstly access brainwave activity that makes the belief in a new reality possible at the neurological level. Once this has been achieved we are in a position to cultivate and cement in an entirely new reality of belief in our ability to recover. The techniques we will be calling upon to facilitate this process include:

1. The use of meditation practices to activate a specific type of brainwave activity called theta waves.

2. The adoption of guided imagery and goal-setting practices to cultivate deep shifts in our reinterpretation of our reality and thus in our ability to then live out this reality.

Over the rest of this chapter, and onwards into the next, we will be discussing each of these practices and exploring how and why they work and how to practically engage in using them. In doing so, you will have a fully evidence-based framework for unleashing the full power of your mind and consciousness and using this in a way that will allow you to thrive in the face of cancer.

## Meditation: Accessing a Place Beyond Cancer

When we say 'I have cancer', this is factually incorrect; the body has cancer, not you. Our mistake is to associate the body with the 'I' inhabiting it. But we are not our body. Nor are we our thoughts. At the base level, our body is simply a field of molecules and our mind a field of thoughts. But beyond these two fields lies another self, our true Self, often called the 'observer'. In the Ayurvedic tradition, this true Self is called *Atman* and it represents perhaps one of the most important components of Vedic philosophy, psychology and spirituality. Atman is the part of you – your purest state of consciousness – that is able to dispassionately observe the workings of both your body and mind as if they belong to someone else.

This sounds abstract but it is very easy to see, and I am sure most people have experience of it. For example, imagine you are stuck in an endless traffic jam and you are getting increasingly agitated and angry. After ten minutes, your anger and frustration feel like they are about to boil over. And yet, even in the intensity of these emotions, there is a part of you that can observe yourself getting angry and frustrated almost like it was happening to someone else. This is a part of you that is separate to and detached from these emotions, a silent witness of them rather than an active participant in them. This observer is your true Self and learning to connect with it is just a matter of practice.

Try this: the next time you are queuing for petrol, stuck in traffic, in a bad mood, feeling stressed or experiencing any other unwanted emotion, step back into your consciousness. Try to connect with the observer that is your true Self and 'watch' yourself experiencing these emotions as if they were happening to someone else. Ask yourself this question: 'Who is getting angry, stressed or frustrated?' Acknowledge that it is just your senses and brain responding to an unwanted event. It is not your true Self as this is beyond the realm of your mind and body. Label the experience. Say to yourself, 'here is me getting angry and frustrated', and smile at the silly and reactive nature of the brain from a place of detachment that is beyond its reach.

Learning to connect with this silent witness frees us from the reactive and often exhausting activity of the monkey mind that is the human brain and instead allows us to use our mind and our consciousness in the empowered pursuit of healing. This process takes practice, but over time it can become our default response to unwanted events and emotions as the brain reconfigures itself (a neurological process called neuroplasticity) in a way that makes such a response a habitual one.

Crucially, this observer that you were trying to identify and connect with in the above task is, by being beyond the body and mind, also beyond the label of cancer, disease, pain and suffering. Indeed, it is beyond everything. Connecting with our true Self in this way moves us from a place of limited, fearful thinking into a place of infinite healing potential. And the more connected we become with this place, the more we harness the limitless healing potential to be found there. This is why virtually every single traditional system of medicine, including Ayurveda, advocates contemplative practices such as meditation as a foundational healing practice in our quest for health. Meditation is the purest way of transcending the self-limiting beliefs of the rational mind (the power of which was so observable in the belief-induced inability of so many athletes to break the four-minute mile for so many years) and moving it instead into a place of limitless possibility in all contexts, including healing.

And yet, unfortunately, the human brain conspires to make this an incredibly difficult thing to achieve. In normal everyday life, when we are working, thinking, analysing, planning, worrying and doing all the millions of other things the mind does during waking state, a part of the brain called the neocortex is dominant. The neocortex is what we associate with our analytical brain or, as it is more commonly known, our ego. It is this ego-dominant state that is largely responsible for the near constant presence of the types of unwanted emotional states that are so common when living with cancer – chronic stress, anxiety, fear, catastrophising and worry, to name but a few.

When the ego-driven analytical mind, and the beta brainwaves it produces, reign supreme, life can feel exhausting. In such a place, cancer, in its broadest sense, can consume us as we obsess over the worst-case scenarios. When this type of mindset is dominant, cultivating genuinely powerful and authentic beliefs around the possibility of becoming exceptional can become incredibly difficult. We become locked in the fear-based brain, a place that restricts open-minded outlooks and resists the view that another alternative is always held open to us: the opportunity of survival. We become like the athletes who, in believing it was impossible for them to break the four-minute mile, made it so. We become self-limiting. This is why it is absolutely imperative that we are able to move beyond the clutches of the neocortex-driven analytical mind and into the limitless potential that is to be found exclusively within the field of human consciousness. And meditation is the vehicle that best gets us there. For in meditation, we are able to access the unique brainwave activity that acts as the neurological key for unlocking the healing powers of the mind.

## Theta Brainwaves and the Gateway to Turiya

If the neocortex-driven beta-brainwave activity represents the rational, analytical and reactive thinking patterns of the fear-based ego, theta brainwaves represent the opposite. Theta brainwaves are associated with the blissful twilight state that we often experience just before falling asleep and are often referred to as our 'healing brainwaves'. In waking conditions, scientific evidence shows us that theta wave activity is also commonly induced by practices such as prayer, silence, solitude, introspection and, of course, meditation.[8] When theta wave activity is dominant, the analytical activity of the brain slows, the ego quietens and we enter a blissful state of oneness and unity.

In the Ayurvedic tradition, this is closely linked to the revered concept of *turiya*. Like Western neurology, Ayurveda recognises the three primary states of consciousness: waking state, dreaming state and deep sleep. However, the Vedic tradition goes one step further and acknowledges a fourth state of consciousness in which all the sense organs are completely retracted from the outside world and our consciousness rests exclusively within our true Self, or Atman. This is turiya. The goal of meditation is to consciously access this state, not just for a few minutes before falling asleep, but in a longer and more empowered way every day. Doing so helps us to build a conscious and subconscious outlook that is beyond the realm of cancer and beyond the ego's fear-based interpretation of it.

Crucially, Western neurological research is now revealing why this shift into theta wave activity is so powerful in the context of mobilising the mechanisms of mind-body healing. More specifically, when in theta wave activity, we are most neurologically suggestible at the subconscious level to new ideas and to the building of new belief systems. The regular activation of theta wave activity can help to reduce the dominance of the ego-driven neocortex and make us far more responsive to the actual, real possibility of a new reality. In other words, cultivating a conscious and subconscious outlook that truly believes in our ability to become exceptional and flourish in the midst of cancer is most powerfully and most effectively done through the regular daily activation of theta brainwave activity. We can think of theta as a controllable mechanism for activating within the neurobiology of the body the same responses that Roger Bannister unlocked in becoming the first person to run the four-minute mile: the actual genuine belief in our ability to achieve it. When in this place, we are then able to more effectively utilise the two additional practices we will explore in the next chapter – namely guided mental imagery and goal setting – to actually and quantifiably alter the neurophysiological workings of the body specific to healing.

In many ways, the analogy of the soil and the seed is a great one here. Even with the best seeds, the growing of a healthy plant requires more than just perfect seeds. It needs optimally prepared and healthy soil. Add strong seeds to healthy soil and the plant will flourish. So it is with the Eastern approaches to mind-body medicine. For practices such as guided imagery and goal setting to work, the soil of the brain must first be prepared. So many times in the past I have seen people working tirelessly to cultivate a genuine belief in their ability to become exceptional, to no avail. Despite their best efforts, their deepest, neocortex-driven beliefs don't shift and they are unable to access that place within them where impossible suddenly transforms into possible. In virtually all these cases, it was because they hadn't prepared the soil of their brain properly. They were trying to build new belief systems while the analytical ego-driven neocortex was still dominant. Until this part of the brain is quietened down, the brain is not neurologically suggestible enough to open up to mobilising the benefits of practices such as guided imagery and goal setting. In contrast, when the ego-driven neocortex is calmed via meditative practices, and the brain is open to a higher level of suggestibility to the cultivation of new belief systems via the regular harnessing of theta brainwaves, the application of these practices can induce profound changes. This is due to the simple fact that the brain neurologically buys into the validity of what it is being fed.

Embedding a regular daily meditation practice in this way can also induce further psychological, emotional and physiological gains for those living with cancer. Over the last twenty years, there has been a veritable explosion of research into the clinical impacts of meditative practices upon the collective health and wellbeing of those living with cancer. And what the collective consensus from this body of research shows is that meditation is a simple, easy and clinically proven modality for effectively reducing stress, anxiety and depression, boosting positive mood states, increasing optimism and enhancing sleep quality in those living with cancer. For example, a study by the Tom Baker Cancer Centre in Alberta, Canada, looked into the effects of mindfulness meditation upon a variety of physical and psychological conditions and assessed how those with cancer using such practices compared to those with cancer who were not using them.[9] The results highlighted that those embedding daily meditation benefited from a 65 per cent reduction in total mood disturbance, including reductions in depression, anxiety and anger. They also felt more vigorous and energised, with reduced levels of daily fatigue, and benefited from a 35 per cent reduction in stress symptoms, including decreased muscle tension and stomach and bowel problems. Crucially, these huge gains were not short lived and transient; they were maintained all the way to the close of the study period six months later, suggesting that as long as the meditation practice is maintained, so too will be the benefits.

Additionally, advances in the field of meditation research have also revealed that regular meditative practice can include clinically significant alterations in physiological variables relevant to cancer survivorship. For example, research undertaken by Linda Witek-Janusek published in the journal *Brain, Behaviour and Immunity*[10] revealed that breast cancer patients using meditation experienced a significant improvement in the activity of their natural killer cells, a type of immune cell that plays a vital role in our anti-cancer defences. The implications of such findings are important because, as the study notes:

Optimal immune function is important for cancer control, especially at times when tumor burden is removed by surgery and immune mechanisms become more essential in defending against any nascent tumor cells. The preponderance of evidence supports the importance of optimal immune function in individuals with cancer. Therefore, interventions that not only reduce psychological stress but also support immune function are advantageous to individuals with cancer.

While the above examples provide just a small snapshot of the available evidence, taken together this research shows just how imperative meditative practices are upon the restoration and optimisation of neurological, immunological, psychological and emotional balance in those living with cancer. As such, the embedding of a daily meditation practice needs to become the cornerstone upon which our collective cancer survivorship framework is built upon.

## How to Meditate: The Practices

The first thing to emphasise about meditation is that we don't need to overcomplicate it. With just a little bit of practise, meditation becomes as simple as breathing. In the sections below I outline three types of meditation practices for you to try. The first is a very simple breath-based practice in which the breath is used as an 'anchor' for your focus. In the second practice, we use a classical Vedic mantra meditation that uses vibrational sound as the anchor. Lastly, we will explore a manualised practice called 'breath balancing', which is a fantastic meditative tool to diffuse high-stress situations, such as when having an MRI or awaiting scan results. For each of these practices there will be a short written guide that you can use to inform your practice. Or, if you would like to be verbally guided through the practice, you can access a free audio download via the links provided in Practice 1 (page 43) and Practice 2 (page 44).

### Preparing for Meditation

Before we begin, it is worth briefly exploring some preparatory concepts that can really help to maximise the effectiveness and long-term sustainability of a daily meditation practice:

## When to Meditate and for How Long?

In terms of when to practise, the simplest answer is whenever is most convenient for you. However, long-term habit formation research shows that we are more likely to embed a practice long term if we complete it at roughly the same time every day (the habitual nature of brushing our teeth is a great example of this). Classically, it is best to make the morning the foundation of your meditation practice; doing so allows you to harness all of the myriad benefits of meditation before your day even begins. For full guidance on how to embed meditation into the Ayurvedic optimal morning routine, please see Self-Developing Practices: Meditation, Journalling and Prayer in chapter 8 (page 153). This brings a discernible level of empowerment, balance, optimism and positivity into the coming day. In terms of duration, this can be fluid: on busy days do less, on quiet days do more. Remember, we don't want to create any sense of friction or stress about undertaking a meditation practice; it needs to feel natural, organic and effortless. But ideally a twenty- to thirty-minute practice in the morning and again in the evening is ideal. Meditation is very much like any other skill; the more time and practice you put in, the easier and more enjoyable it becomes.

## Where to Meditate

As with deciding when and for how long to meditate, keeping things simple is important here and the best answer is anywhere and everywhere. On a warm sunny day, you might want to take your practice into the garden. On a cold winter's day, you might practise in bed under the warmth of a blanket. However, that said, there is something incredibly empowering and energising about having a designated meditation spot, whether this is a spare room, a corner of a room, a garden office or any other nook or cranny you can dedicate to your practice.

In this space, you can decorate how you like; perhaps hang inspiring pictures or quotes on the wall, fill it with beautiful flowers and aromas, buy a sacred meditation mat or cushion or add any other personal touches that will make you feel calm and relaxed in that special place. Personally speaking, I have found having a specific location like this to be of immense value; just walking into my meditation room induces a sense of peace and calm before I even begin. This space can also be used for other self-care pursuits, such as yoga, journalling or reading, or simply as a bolthole to escape the demands of everyday life for a while.

## Practice 1: Breath-Based Meditation

It usually helps to practise meditation in a comfortable, straight-backed chair or sitting on the floor, adopting a dignified and erect posture but one that is as comfortable as possible. Try to have your feet flat on the floor, or cross your legs if sitting on the floor, with your hands open on your lap in whatever position feels most natural. Most people find it easiest to meditate with their eyes closed and I suggest you try this approach first. If you find sitting like this uncomfortable for any reason, then you can just as effectively meditate lying down. In this case, support your head with a pillow and keep your legs and ankles uncrossed and your hands on your thigh area. It is very easy to fall asleep when lying this way but try to resist this! Just make sure that you are comfortable in whatever position you are in and that you are wearing loose, relaxing clothes.

To begin the meditation, simply take three to four very deep and slow diaphragmatic in-breaths and out-breaths, aiming to completely fill and empty the lungs as you do so. This is a great way to calm the mind and body in preparation for meditation. Then, slowly let your breathing return to its normal rhythm. Now, bring your awareness onto your breath, which will act as the 'anchor' of your attention. As you breathe in, hold your attention on the sensations of air moving into your lungs and your expanding abdomen. Really try to feel and deeply connect with these physical sensations. Then, as you breathe out, hold your awareness on your tummy as it contracts and the sensation of air moving up from your lungs and out of your nostrils. Then, as you breathe in again, repeat this process in such a way that your entire field of awareness holds on to the alternating physical experience of breathing in and breathing out. Set a timer with a gentle and soothing alarm and aim to stay in this meditation for twenty to thirty minutes. A full twenty-five-minute audio-guided breath-based meditation is included under Guided Meditations in the online resources for this book, which can be accessed at www.mind-body-medical.co.uk/becomingexceptional.

## Practice 2: Vedic Mantra Meditation

In this practice, we use the same technique as used in Practice 1, but this time, rather than using the breath as the anchor of our awareness, we use a mantra. A mantra is a verbal concentration aid that we use during meditation to slow the workings of the rational brain and to support deeper contemplative states. One of the most famous and revered Vedic mantras, and a great one to start with, is the 'om' mantra. In the Vedic tradition, the sound om is regarded as the initial vibration that brought all things in the universe into existence. It is for this reason that om is referred to as the 'cosmic sound' and is viewed as a sacred sound with powerful healing potential.

To use this manta, take a slow and controlled in-breath, and then on the out-breath, place all your awareness on creating the sound om (pronounced 'ommm'). This should be experienced as a humming sound that creates a deep vibration all along the back of the mouth and throat. Then simply repeat this process of taking a slow and controlled in-breath followed by the repetition of the om mantra on the out-breath. My experience of this meditation is that it invokes a profoundly deep sense of calm and relaxation in which time passes incredibly quickly and we emerge from the meditation feeling revitalised and powerful. Access to a twenty-five-minute guided mantra meditation can also be found in the Guided Meditations section of the online resources found at www.mind-body-medical.co.uk/becomingexceptional.

### Practice 3: Breath Balancing

This is a fantastically helpful form of meditation that excels in deactivating acute stress. There are a whole host of situations that are commonplace for those living with cancer, such as awaiting results, during scans and the prospect of invasive procedures, that can all invoke often debilitating levels of stress. Having tools to manage these kinds of acute stressors is therefore incredibly important. And in that capacity, breath-balancing meditations excel. This is because they allow us to consciously activate a part of our nervous system called the parasympathetic nervous system (PNS), which is responsible for activating the rest, heal and digest mechanisms of our body. In other words, they activate the relaxation response and through doing so lower stress levels.

This is in direct contrast with our sympathetic nervous system (SNS), which is responsible for activating the body's stress response, often referred to as our fight or flight response. When we are facing an acute stressor such as those mentioned above, our PNS is deactivated as our SNS kicks in, leading to the all too common physical and emotional responses we experience when stressed. However, if we are able to suppress the SNS and activate the PNS during such situations, we can make a discernible impact upon lowering the levels of stress we experience. And what the evidence shows is that when we extend or prolong the exhalation phase of our breath cycle, it induces a significant activation of the PNS. Thus, if we consciously breathe in a way that focuses on embedding a pause after the out-breath, we can 'trick' the nervous system into switching off the stress response in favour of activating the relaxation response.

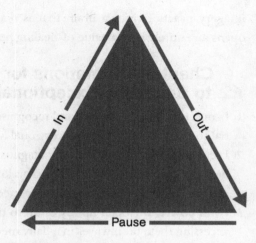

Figure 3.3. The triangle of conscious breathing.

To practise this technique, visualise in your mind an equally sided triangle. Starting at the bottom left-hand corner of the triangle, inhale deeply for a specified count (usually three to four seconds) and then immediately exhale for the same length of time. After the exhalation has ended, pause for a count of four seconds before beginning the process again with the next in-breath. Each phase of the breathing pattern (in-breath, out-breath, pause) represents one side of the triangle, and it can be very helpful to visualise in your mind your breath travelling along this triangle as you count, as referenced in figure 3.3. The next time you find yourself experiencing an acute stress response, this is a fantastic technique to turn to.

---

Now that we have explored why meditation is such a foundationally important practice to embed in the context of cancer survivorship, the priority is to actually integrate it into your daily life until it becomes habitual. By doing this, we begin to harness all the physical and emotional benefits that come with it. Even more so, it will ensure the daily activation of theta wave activity, which, as we have seen, is a neurological prerequisite for increasing the brain's suggestibility to the possibility of a new reality relevant to healing. In the next chapter, we will explore how combining a selection of guided imagery practices into a brain that is neurologically suggestible to them opens an entirely new avenue of healing potential.

## 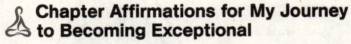 Chapter Affirmations for My Journey to Becoming Exceptional

1. I consciously acknowledge and recognise the inherent and infinite potential to survive and become exceptional lying within me.
2. I recognise that others with my diagnosis and prognosis have gone on to become exceptional and I will use this knowledge to cultivate deep within me the belief that I too can become exceptional.
3. I will powerfully open up my brain to the possibility of new realities via accessing theta brainwaves in a daily meditation practice.
4. **Summary Affirmation:** Each and every day I nourish my mind as I engineer my own reality on my journey to becoming exceptional.

# CHAPTER FOUR

# Onwards to Imagery
## The Recreation of Reality

> *Reality is how we interpret it. Imagination and volition play a part in that interpretation. Which means that all reality is to some extent a fiction.*
>
> YANN MARTEL

Now that we have explored why meditation is so important and how it alters the neurobiology of the brain in a way that increases its suggestibility to the possibility of new realities, it is time to actually create those realities. And to do that we need to turn to the mind-bending research and mechanisms of guided imagery, visualisation and, as strange as it sounds, quantum mechanics. But firstly, what is guided imagery?

In its simplest form, it is the process of creating mental images around a desired outcome of a future event in a way that maximises the chances of that outcome reaching fruition. Today, the professional application of guided imagery exists squarely in the mainstream; NASA uses it to best prepare their astronauts, Formula One racing champions use intense guided imagery before each race to create the perfect execution of their performance and concert pianists routinely use guided imagery to speed up the learning of complex symphonies and the finger placements needed to play them properly. In other words, a desired reality is firstly imagined and visualised in the mind before it manifests as a physical reality in the world. In such instances, the impacts and benefits afforded by imagery extend far beyond the realm of just positive thinking; they go on to directly alter the physiological workings of the body. Consider these words from Denis Waitley, who cemented the use of guided imagery in the US Olympic programme:

Using imagery, the Olympic athletes ran their event in their minds. They imagined how they looked and felt when they were actually participating in their event. The athletes were then hooked up to a sophisticated biofeedback machine, and its results told the real story about the value of imagery. The same muscles fired in the same sequence as when they were actually running on the track! This proved that the mind can't tell the difference between whether you're really doing something or whether you are imagining doing it. If you've been there in the mind, you'll go there in the body.[1]

However, the crucial point for us is that in the same way that guided imagery can cause muscles to fire in the desired way, it can also alter a whole host of other physiological variables relevant to healing and cancer survivorship, such as immune activity,[2] sleep quality and pain management.[3] Paradigm-changing research has shown that it may even be causally linked to longer survival times in those with terminal cancer, as we shall explore below.[4] And it is only right that imagery should be as effective in the context of healing as it is in the context of enhancing athletic performance; African shamans, Himalayan monks and the towering early physicians of ancient Greece, such as Hippocrates and Galen, all turned to imagery and visualisation practices as a tool to induce healing. So, too, in Ayurveda, which puts significant emphasis on the practice of *sankalpa*.

Sankalpa is the conscious creation of sacred intentions and visualisations that provide us with a vehicle for mobilising the power of our mind in the realisation of our highest dreams, ideals and goals, including the recovery from illness and the cultivation of our highest levels of health. These days, imagery is listed in the top ten most popular complementary practices used by those with cancer, is endorsed by leading cancer research centres, such as the American Cancer Society, and has been adopted into the integrative practices of the world's leading cancer hospitals, such as the Mayo Clinic in the US.

However, prior to the 1970s the clinical application of guided imagery in the Western healthcare arena was very much on the fringe and was still viewed with much suspicion. That was all to change when the concept of guided imagery piqued the interest of American radiation oncologist Dr O. Carl Simonton. And the research he published around the use of guided imagery specifically in the context of cancer survivorship not only opened the doors for the wholesale adoption of such practices in the field of integrative cancer care. It also rocked the established medical understanding of the potential of the human body to overcome advanced cancers and how imagery and visualisation practices can be used to harness and optimise this potential.

## The Move Into Medicine: Guided Imagery and Exceptional Cancer Survival

The entire field of integrative cancer survivorship owes a true dept of gratitude to Dr O. Carl Simonton. For this trailblazing clinician was open-minded enough to acknowledge the limitations of conventional cancer management and explore how mind-body practices could be used to antidote these limitations. More specifically, what Dr Simonton recognised early in his career as an oncologist was that despite having the same diagnoses, prognoses and treatment, those with cancer who maintained a sense of optimism, positivity and hope consistently lived longer and in better health than those who didn't.

This led to him diving into the research and mechanisms of mind-body medicine and ultimately to the discovery of the central, integral role played by imagery and visualisation. He soon established his own cancer treatment centre (the Simonton Cancer Center), which blended the best of both conventional and mind-body cancer care into one model. The results he obtained were incredible and his patients consistently outlived and outperformed those with the same disease not using his methods. Encouraged by his early success, he went on to publish his seminal book *Getting Well Again*.

This book was Dr Simonton's magnum opus and, so many decades later, should still be regarded as mandatory reading for those living with cancer. In it, he discusses the clinically validated ability of guided imagery to actually and quantifiably alter human physiology, and in some cases prolong survival in those with incurable cancers. More specifically, he reported data from a four-year study of 159 patients with medically incurable cancer who were treated exclusively by Dr Simonton using his Simonton Method. The medical records of all these patients were independently reviewed by a panel of oncologists and their collective view was that none of them could be expected to survive for more than twelve months based on their clinical profiles. At the end of the four-year study period, the results were as follows:

- 22.2 per cent of patients showed *no signs of disease* and had made a full and impossible recovery.

- 19.1 per cent of patients experienced a clinically significant reduction of their disease.
- 27.1 per cent of patients experienced stable disease with no signs of growth.
- 31.8 per cent of patients experienced disease progression.

This study and the incredible results it presents to us are now so famous that there is a risk that we skim past them without really meditating on their significance and relevance. If we keep in mind that *all* these individuals were considered to be medically incurable and that none of them were predicted to survive for more than twelve months, these results are paradigm changing. And while it is of vital importance that we don't fall into the trap of simplifying these results to suggest that guided imagery can cure cancer (which it can't), what they do suggest is that the regular practice of mind-body techniques such as guided imagery can induce profound changes in the physiology of the body that are vital for us to harness in our quest to become exceptional.

It is also important to emphasise that this research does not stand in isolation. Dr Simonton very much sowed the seeds of the use of guided imagery in the arena of cancer. But in the ensuing decades, these seeds have blossomed into the large and growing foundation of clinical research that we benefit from today. There are now dozens upon dozens of peer-reviewed, published clinical studies showing that in those living with cancer, guided imagery can positively impact upon a whole host of variables specific to cancer survivorship, such as improved immune function, enhanced psychological wellbeing,[5] reduced levels of pain, fatigue, anxiety and nausea and much else besides.[6] Given the strength of this research, the application of regular guided imagery needs to inform a key aspect of a fully integrative and evidence-based cancer survivorship protocol.

## Types of Imagery

While there are myriad ways of using imagery to target everything from sleep quality and stress reduction to pain management and immune modulation, in the rest of this chapter I want to focus on two specific and particularly important types: 1) envisioning health imagery; and 2) goal-setting imagery. Due to the vastly different objectives, mechanisms and techniques inherent in these two different practices, they are each explored individually.

## *Imagery Practice 1: Envisioning Health*

Envisioning health imagery is the most physiologically active form of guided imagery and the one that has arguably received the most research focus over the last few decades. The practice involves the process of creating detailed mental images of your immune system effectively and efficiently identifying, targeting and destroying any cancer cells in your body, as visualised in your mind's eye. As the guided practice progresses, you begin to generate, with as much vivid accuracy as possible, detailed mental imagery of individual cancer cells being destroyed and whole tumours being systematically broken down and removed from the body. This process is continued until, towards the end of the practice, you visualise the end-goal you are striving to realise: your body being completely free of all cancer burden and your body operating in a place of radical health.

This was the type of visualisation that was initially developed and promoted by Dr Simonton in his research cited previously and the type that has been most widely applied in the context of cancer. The physiological mechanisms that this type of imagery is able to induce relevant to its ability to alter the workings of the body in the direction of healing are now clearly and evidentially documented. And it all starts in a part of the brain called the frontal lobe. This area of the brain is a primary seat of consciousness and is largely responsible for goal setting, creative thinking, problem solving and decision making. Crucially, when engaged in guided imagery practices, it is the frontal lobe that is primarily called to action. This is important because when the frontal lobe is dominant in this way, we often lose our sense of the 'outside' world and also of our basic needs such as eating, drinking and even the passing of time. If you think back to any time in your life when you were so engaged in something – a book, a film, painting, music or a hobby – that you lost all sense of anything other than the pursuit you were partaking in, this is frontal lobe dominance. Because our focus on the 'outside' world is diminished, the reality of our 'inner world' moves into sharper focus and any visualisations, goals or intentions we focus on become much starker and real. This is why the detail and accuracy of the imagery we create is of such importance; it has to essentially trick the brain into believing it is real.

At this point, once the assessment by the frontal lobe is that the imagery being generated is valid and real, it gets to work to turn the observed reality (i.e. the imagery you are creating) into a physical response in the body. To do this, it calls upon the now famous neuropeptides that we briefly discussed in The Ayurvedic View and Understanding of Cancer in chapter 2 (page 18). Remember, neuropeptides are our molecules of emotion that allow our thoughts, feelings and beliefs to directly interact with and modulate the action of the cells found within our body. When using guided imagery to imagine the process of your immune system effectively identifying and destroying cancer cells, the brain creates neuropeptides in direct response to the images you have been working with. These neuropeptides are then sent out to dock onto the neuropeptide receptor sites of the body's immune cells. Once they have docked onto the immune cells, they deliver the chemical message they carry directly to the DNA found within the immune cells, which in turn goes on to directly alter immune activity. Given that this message is to tell the immune cells to behave in a way that allows them to more effectively target and destroy cancer cells, we can now see why there is such compelling evidence to show how guided imagery practices can induce such significant improvements in immune function, particularly in those with cancer.

While such mechanisms can appear quite complex, we can best see them play out in the more commonplace example of our televisions. Neurologically speaking, images observed on a screen are absolutely no different to images created by the brain; what the brain sees it responds to, irrespective of whether the images are created from within or from without. So, when we watch a film that is scary or intimidating or movingly sad, what happens? We experience an observable physiological response. If it is a terrifying horror show, we get nervous, anxious, our heart rate goes up and, at the base level, we feel scared. Why? Our rational brain knows it is a fictious film. We know the characters are actors working on a film set with a director, make-up artists and a coffee machine. But none of this matters. We see something scary, the brain reacts to what it sees and our body responds. So, too, with healing imagery; it is a purely cause–effect relationship. We just simply need to create enough detail, accuracy and vividness in the imagery we create to ensure the frontal lobe buys into it. If we can do that, all subsequent responses are simply a chain reaction until the end result – enhanced immune activity – is observed.

## The Practice
When sitting down to start guided imagery, the same preparatory guidelines mentioned for Practice 1 in the previous chapter apply. However, guided

imagery scripts, such as those used in the envisioning health practice, are detailed and extensive, so I have included a full written guide for practising this technique in appendix 2 (page 223). If you are new to guided imagery, it is often easier to be verbally guided through the practice, so you will also find there a link to a free audio download to help get you started in the most effective way possible.

## Imagery Practice 2:
## Creating the Future Now – Goal-Setting Imagery

Having explored the envisioning health imagery, we can now turn our attention to the final practice of this chapter, goal-setting imagery. This practice is a crucially important one and one that I have used and prioritised with virtually every single person with cancer I have ever worked with. It is also a fascinating practice that joins together the ancient spiritual and philosophical teachings of Ayurveda with the most advanced understanding of quantum mechanics to explain how goal setting, visualisation and intention has the potential to tangibly alter the physical reality of our lives. The entire aim and focus of goal-setting imagery is to visualise, in great detail, our future lives and all the deeply meaningful dreams, goals and experiences we want to realise in it.

This isn't about creating a bucket list of things we want to achieve in a short period of time before we die. Rather it is an immensely powerful projection of a healthy, happy and meaningful life that extends years into the future and what our priorities are for using that time in the richest way possible. It is about moving our awareness beyond the realm of cancer and imprinting into the conscious and subconscious mind the actual tangible reality of a long and healthy life.

Think deeply about what your goals, dreams and ambitions were before your cancer diagnosis. These dreams need to take on an even greater level of meaning subsequent to your diagnosis than they ever did before it. Plan these dreams, prepare for them and expect to realise them with unquestioning faith. Doing so, over time, imprints into our consciousness the belief that these dreams will happen, irrespective of any statistics you may be facing. One of the criticisms I often encounter when talking about these types of practices is that they run the risk of proffering false hope. This is a misnomer. There is either hope or there isn't. And as long as there is breath in our bodies then there is hope. And perhaps more than any other quality, it is hope that we need to most powerfully and proactively cultivate into our lives, especially when all hope seems to be lost.

Over the years, I have had the privilege of seeing so many inspiring individuals, such as Janet, whom we met in the introduction to this book, who have ridden into the realm of exceptional on the back of hope. When we live with hope – hope of seeing our children or grandchildren leave school, build happy lives and get married, hope of travelling to far-flung exotic locations, hope of realising meaningful goals, hope of reaching key life milestones – it lights a fire in our being that fuels a completely new shift in our outlook. Dreaming of these 'hopes' no longer leaves us feeling sad and grief-filled because we think we will never get to realise them. Rather, it leaves us feeling excited, optimistic and empowered because we realise that we do have the ability to realise them and, more importantly, that we will.

Goal-setting imagery, then, is a technique that requires as much proactive work and focus as any other survivorship tool. As we shall see, the Ayurvedic tradition and the modern world of quantum mechanics mechanistically agree upon the fact that these types of practices have the capacity to alter the workings of the physical universe around us in a way that allows the dreams and goals we are visualising to reach tangible fruition. If that sounds a little far-fetched, what we'll explore next might surprise you.

## Ayurveda, The Unified Field and Quantum Theory

I appreciate that a move into the arena of quantum theory may seem a little abstract in a book dealing with exceptional cancer survivorship. But at the most profound level, it isn't, and it is absolutely essential that we all understand why. Because with a deeper understanding of quantum theory, we begin to truly grasp just why goal-setting imagery is so vitally important. With this grasped, the motivation to engage and comply with such practices will be greatly enhanced. And in doing so, we unlock the infinite potential for healing and transformation to be found there. So in the following sections, I want to briefly discuss this topic from the perspective of both classical Ayurveda and Western quantum physics before exploring the actual practice itself.

In the Vedic tradition, there is a beautifully simple concept that is also, paradoxically, infinitely complex. It is this: 'I am that, you are that, all this is that, and that is all there is.' In other words, everything in physical existence, from stars and galaxies to human beings, oceans and seashells, were all originally manifested from the same source. And that source was a conscious and intelligent primordial energy that existed before all matter was manifested. In the Vedic tradition, this is called the 'akashic field', which can be equated to the concept of the Minkowski vacuum in quantum physics. From this field of pure potentiality, a sudden and rapid expansion of space itself occurred, the outcome of which was what we now call the Big Bang – the seismic galactic event from which everything in physical existence emerged. It is for this reason that in Vedic philosophy, the akashic field is regarded as the foundation of the material world in which we live. But, from the perspective of both Ayurveda and quantum physics, this physical matter is not matter at all, but rather vibrational energy. In the physical sense, everything in material existence, from your body to the chair you are sitting on, is made up of atoms, which are the building blocks of all matter in the universe. But as quantum physicists began to explore the structure of the atom in greater detail, ever smaller subatomic particles were discovered until, as they continued looking, all physical and tangible matter disappeared. So much so that it is now an accepted scientific fact that atoms are made up of 99.9999999 per cent empty space. Which, extrapolated out, means everything in physical existence, including your body, also comprises 99.9999999 per cent empty space because your body is simply an accumulation of atoms. This is not theoretical conjecture but the highest and most advanced level of scientific evidence.[7]

However, as these pioneering physicists kept on probing the secrets of the atom, an even more important fact emerged. They discovered that this 99.9999999 per cent nothingness isn't actually nothing. Rather, it is made up of unimaginably concentrated vibrating energy. Which again is to say that every physical thing in existence, including our bodies, is also made up almost exclusively of energy. Why is this important? Because the most astonishing discovery they made was that the subatomic matter found within the atom could exist as either a physical particle with mass and matter or it could exist as pure energy without mass or matter. In other words, it could either exist as particle energy or wave energy.

But this is the crux: what dictates whether a subatomic particle behaves as a physical particle or as an energy wave is the now famous 'observer effect'. More specifically, whenever the scientists put their conscious attention on any one electron in their attempt to study it, that electron instantly appeared in physical particle form. But as soon as they took their attention off it, the reverse occurred and it instantly disappeared back into pure wave energy. This observer effect is now a fundamental concept within the field of quantum physics and its implications are profound. Because what it means is that virtually all matter exists as vibrating wave energy until it is manifested into physical particle energy. At the most foundational level, this manifestation is brought into tangible and observable reality by the placing of conscious attention onto it. In the truest sense, this is the science of mind making matter at the atomic level. And because these subatomic particles don't follow the normal rules of time and space, they can appear in an infinite number of possible ways and locations at any one time. Thus, at the subatomic level, every possible outcome always exists as pure potential. But what occurs – the event or reality that actually plays out in front of us – is dependent upon where we put our attention. For example, if a scientist studying subatomic particles put her attention on one particular location, the particle she was studying would appear specifically in that location in time and space. But if she had chosen to put her attention in a different location, the same particle would have appeared there. Both outcomes existed as pure potential but the one that actually occurred was dictated by where her attention was placed.

In light of these findings, we can accept as scientific fact that at the level of energy – which makes up 99.999999 per cent of everything in existence, including us – every possible outcome exists as a potential quantum reality. And we have the capacity to collapse this infinite quantum potential into a specific and chosen outcome via the placing of conscious energy upon it. When you use detailed, creative imagery in this way to envision a future outcome – the regaining of optimal health, recovery from disease, realising long-term goals or any other meaningful outcome – that reality already exists somewhere at the quantum level as a potential outcome. And in the same way that the conscious placing of attention can manifest the appearance of an electron into physical reality, at the quantum level it is also theoretically possible for us to influence the appearance of a future reality we aspire to.

It is for this reason that imagery and visualisation practices are so powerful at bringing about change. If you are able to create in your mind incredible detailed and emotionally driven imagery scripts of a future you want to experience, at the level of your consciousness you would actually be inhabiting that future event right now because, neurologically speaking, a detailed image of a future event seen in great detail is just as real as an actual image observed in the here and now.

The more time we spend imagining and envisioning this future, ultimately the more attention we put onto it. And remember, at the level of quantum theory, every possible outcome exists in every moment as the energy of potential. What informs whether that potential reaches actual physical fruition is the level and intensity of the attention we put on it. So, by consciously placing our attention on the future reality you are aiming for via the practice of guided imagery, you drastically increase the chance of that reality maturing into physical reality. To further support the scientific validity of this concept, we can turn to one of the most influential quantum physicists of all time, Max Planck. Professor Planck was a German theoretical physicist who won the Nobel Prize in 1918 for the first discovery of energy quanta. From this lofty position among the upper echelon of academic achievements, his now famous quote takes on even greater significance:

> As a man who has devoted his whole life to the most clearheaded science, to the study of matter, I can tell you as a result of my research about the atoms this much: There is no matter as such! All matter originates and exists only by virtue of a force which brings the particles of an atom to vibration and holds this most minute solar system of the atom together. We must assume behind this force the existence of a conscious and intelligent mind. Mind is the matrix of all matter.[8]

Goal-setting imagery should not be viewed as weak and unscientific wishful thinking but rather as the 'matrix of all matter' and as a tool for manifesting our future goals and dreams at the most fundamental level of physical reality: the level of energy. Remember, 'where attention goes, energy flows', and by consciously placing our attention onto what we want to happen, we will be affecting matter in a profound way. We saw an example of this in the work of Dr Simonton, which we discussed in The Move Into Medicine on page 49. More specifically, it was observed that patients who went on to do very well and far surpass their prognosis:

- had very strong goals that they wanted to achieve
- could elaborate on these goals in great detail
- felt an intense attachment to these goals

In addition to quantum mechanics, Dr Simonton elaborated on the benefits of goal-setting imagery in three key areas. Setting and visualising the fruition of goals:

- tells your mind that you fully expect to make a complete recovery
- reaffirms that you are in control of your life
- provides a focus for your energy

**Practising Goal-Setting Imagery**

Unlike the envisioning health imagery, it is not possible to create generic guided imagery scripts for goal-setting imagery. This is because for the latter to work effectively, it needs to be powerfully individualised and deeply meaningful to the person using it. In the sections below, I have outlined some strategies for facilitating this. However, before exploring these, arguably the most effective means of describing how this process works is to look at someone who actually used this technique effectively in their journey to becoming exceptional. And Penny is a great example of this.

I first met Penny at a cancer survivorship programme I was running at a National Health Service integrative cancer care centre. She was living with terminal stage 4 breast cancer with a prognosis of one to two years. Penny was an incredibly positive and upbeat woman who, in her own words, had a lot of living left to do. And when, during the group sessions, we got to the modules around goal-setting imagery, she was positively bursting to tell the group about hers. This was because, ever since she was in her twenties, she had wanted to walk all the lakeside hiking paths in the Lake District National Park in England. However, full-time work, followed by marriage and then children, had never allowed enough time for Penny to realise this dream. And it was a regret she carried with her. However, in her own words, 'One of the good things to come out of my cancer journey was that it motivated me to re-evaluate my life and reconnect with this dream to walk the Lake District trails.'

Realising that now was the time to act on this goal, she set to work making it a reality. That began with the very practical need to organise the logistics of such an undertaking, including ordering the walking guides, buying new hiking boots, starting a walking-based fitness programme and booking accommodation. (All of which further emphasised to her conscious and subconscious mind that she fully expected these goals to reach fruition.) But in addition to these very practical tasks, she also initiated with unwavering commitment an extensive daily imagery practice. And one of the reasons I chose Penny for this case study was the success she had with her imagery. Every day she would retreat to her bedroom, dim the lights and initiate her goal-setting imagery. Specifically, she would imagine it was the very last day of her adventure and the very last mile of the 125 miles she had thus far walked in undertaking this dream. And she walked that last mile in her mind with the same level of detail and accuracy as if she were actually there. She saw her boots, covered in mud, scuffed and scraped and well and truly broken in. She saw the slightly muddy path she was following, the vibrant green of the summer grass, the sensation of a gentle wind in her face, the location of the sun, the weight of the backpack on her shoulders, her husband next to her and the sheer delicious delight of realising her goal. She physically engineered these emotions in her body and mind during her imagery; the sense of achievement, joy and happiness and a deep inner conviction in her ability to overcome any obstacle. She imagined walking that last mile, step by step, until the path ended at a traditional tearoom on the lake shore. She imagined walking into that tearoom, and the warmth, the smells, the sight of the cakes, the décor and the table she sat at, the steaming pot of tea, the scone and jam. Then the taxi back to their hotel, the joy of a hot shower and an evening basking in her achievements. Finally, she ended the imagery back at her own home in the south of England, planning her next goal in full and vibrant health.

This imagery took her between twenty and thirty minutes every day but this was contemplative time she eagerly looked forward to. It empowered her with the unique ability to create her own future rather than having it dictated to her. The last time I was in contact with Penny, she was doing well and was soon to be off on her next adventure walking the Italian lakes. And while there are obviously myriad factors that are responsible for Penny's incredible move into exceptional – including her conventional cancer treatments and the complementary approaches she was adhering to – I strongly believe that her steadfast commitment to her goal, and the daily visualisation of it, was one of the most important. Penny's story brings into sharp focus the key variables that are needed for goal-setting imagery to work: clarity of the goal, an emotional connection with that goal, the ability to create phenomenally detailed imagery around the completion of the goal and an unwavering commitment to daily imagery practice of the realisation of the goal. The following sections provide guidance for empowering you to do likewise.

## How to Develop an Effective Goal-Setting Imagery Practice

Developing a goal-setting imagery practice is a twofold process. Firstly, it is about spending time identifying and developing your goals on a variety of levels over a variety of time frames. Secondly, it is about spending quality time imagining yourself achieving these goals in great detail. Both of these stages are overviewed next.

### IDENTIFYING AND SETTING GOALS

To practise goal-setting imagery, you firstly need to identify a goal, or goals. In my experience, the best way to do this is from a place of deep contemplation and quietude. Find the time and space to be alone for a full day and reflect deeply and emotionally on your life, the things you love to do, the things you have always wanted to do but as yet haven't; your hobbies, passions and interests. From these thoughts begin to put together an overview of your goals. The more emotionally driven and meaningful these goals are, the more effective they will be. Buying a lovely journal that you use exclusively for these kinds of practices, including those explored later in this book, is strongly recommended. In this you can write down your thoughts, unload emotions and get clarity on your goals; doing so makes them much more tangible and real and therefore much harder to forget and ignore.

### TIME FRAMES

The next important issue to address is the differing time frames of your goals. It is not very helpful having all your goals five years away as this is often too far away to excite and motivate you in the short term. Likewise, you also don't want to set all of your goals in the next six months because that is not looking far ahead enough into the future. It is often best to have a mixture of goals over a five-year time frame that include those that are obtainable over the next six months, one year, three years and five years. This is obviously dependent upon each person's individual circumstances and the time frames can vary hugely. The key thing to remember is to create and list goals that cover a prolonged period of time (from six months through to five years and beyond). In doing so, you have goals to look forward to and motivate you in the short term but are also aware of the 'bigger picture' and the fact that you are reaffirming to your conscious and subconscious mind, not to mention the quantum field, your unshakeable belief in your ability to physically realise goals a long way into the future.

## MAKE YOUR GOALS CONCRETE AND SPECIFIC

It is very important that the goals you set are specific and not vague. Research very much shows that when we set vague goals they are very rarely achieved. In Penny's example, she inherently realised the importance of moving away from a loosely defined 'I am going to walk each of the lakes' to 'I am going to walk each of the lakes, and this is how I am going to do it'. She then set a very logical and achievable set of smaller goals, which I've listed here, that would allow her to reach her overall goal:

> I am going to increase my daily walking to two hours a day, carrying a backpack.
> I will buy hill-walking boots and break them in.
> I will buy a guidebook to the Lake District and plan my route.
> I will create a timetable of when I plan to start.
> I will research and book accommodation.
> I will ensure I am fit enough by the start date to achieve this goal.

This approach gives you the satisfaction of ticking off each mini-goal as and when you achieve it, meaning you are moving closer towards the overall goal. Lastly, don't fall into the trap of making all your goals 'significant'. In my experience, some of the most effective and uplifting goals include simple things like driving to a beautiful place for a picnic on a regular basis with those you love the most, learning to paint or travelling to a long-dreamed-of holiday location.

Once you have your goals identified over a variety of time frames, you need to regularly spend time creating vivid and detailed imagery of yourself achieving those goals. There is no right or wrong way of creating goal-setting imagery. The important thing to remember is to create as much vivid detail in the imagery as possible, as we saw in Penny's example. As with all these techniques, always go with what feels correct to you in terms of how you generate your imagery and in what sequence. However, in my experience it is often easier to start the imagery with the end results (i.e. reaching your goal) and then work backwards to see how you got there. Try using this approach, and if you don't get on with it, give your mind free rein and develop a goal-setting imagery approach that feels right for you.

1. Start your imagery session by selecting one of your specific goals and then visualise yourself achieving that goal in as much detail as possible.

2. Imagine what it would feel like when you reach that goal – emotionally and physically; what emotions would it evoke, how would you feel? The more emotion you attach to the imagery, the greater the impact.
3. Who would be with you when you reach the goal? How would they react? What would you do afterwards? Where would you be?
4. In every aspect of the imagery, really try to evoke as much detail as possible: imagine colours, noises, the location, the atmosphere, the environment.
5. Then work backwards and list the stages you need to go through to achieve that goal (see the Lake District example in Make Your Goals Concrete and Specific on page 61)
6. Finally, imagine yourself reaching and ticking off those stages.

Get creative with this process. Realise and acknowledge the infinite potential for healing and transformation that lies within your mind and your imagery, right down to the quantum level, and commit to harnessing this on a daily basis via a structured imagery practice. After just a short period of time, your belief in the future, and your ability to realise it, soars and with that will always come an increased level of energy, vitality, optimism and, at base, healing.

##  Chapter Affirmations for My Journey to Becoming Exceptional

1. I consciously acknowledge and recognise the power of guided imagery as a tool for transforming the physical health and functioning of my body specific to cancer survivorship.
2. Similarly, I consciously acknowledge the importance and power of goal-setting imagery as a tool for creating the future of my dreams in my body and my larger life.
3. I commit to contemplatively exploring my dreams and using these to fuel an excitement and optimism for the future in the knowledge that I can and will see these dreams reach physical fruition.
4. I commit to embedding a regular guided imagery practice that will best allow me to harness the full and complete benefits it affords.
5. **Summary Affirmation:** Each and every day I commit to unleashing the full power of guided mental imagery as a vital tool in my journey to becoming exceptional.

# CHAPTER FIVE

# Laying Strong Foundations
## *Ayurvedic Anti-Cancer Nutrition*

> *When diet is correct, medicine is of no need. When diet is incorrect, medicine is of no use.*
>
> CHARAKA, *Charaka Samhita*

In our quest to thrive in the face of cancer and progress along the road to becoming exceptional, dietary modification and optimisation is essential. In her internationally best-selling book *Radical Remission*, Kelly A. Turner highlights dietary modification as being one of the nine most commonplace practices adopted by those people living with cancer who go on to become exceptional. This is a view mirrored in the Ayurvedic tradition, which places immense importance upon the therapeutic value of diet in the cultivation of robust health and the management of disease. And when it comes to harnessing the therapeutic potential of our diet in this way, we need to learn to view what we eat through a completely different lens: the lens of medicine. Because every mouthful of food we eat, with the right knowledge, has the capacity to activate profound healing mechanisms in the body. And these mechanisms are accumulative and exponential as the levels of therapeutically active compounds in the body begin to build up over time. For this reason, the optimisation of our diet in a systematic way is of immense importance in the field of cancer survivorship.

This is a view now validated by robust clinical evidence that highlights the potential of myriad plant-based nutrients, compounds and chemicals to suppress virtually all the primary mechanisms that cancer uses to promote growth.[1] Our task is to learn how to harness this potential, not just occasionally or regularly, but every day. All of us have to eat and most of us eat multiple times each day, and the impact of our food choices leaves no room for subjective interpretation: food is either healing or harming. There are very few grey areas, particularly in the context of anti-cancer nutrition. Our challenge is to ensure that our default setting is the consumption of nutrient-dense food that is specifically orientated around the suppression of cancer cell biology.

Viewed in this light we can see why the explosion of cancer-specific nutritional research over the last three decades is so incredibly important; it is motivating and empowering and offers real hope in the broader arena of cancer survivorship. However, this explosion of research has in many ways created its own problem. The sheer variety of different diets, approaches and recommendations available to us makes it incredibly difficult to know where to start when it comes to optimising our own diet in the face of cancer. Particularly as so much of this information is fragmented, disjointed and very difficult to implement in a coherent and practical way. There is no 'unified framework of nutrition' that we can call upon to guide what we should be eating in a way that ensures there are no oversights or weaknesses in such choices. Furthermore, much of the available research remains confined within the sphere of academic medicine, scientific journals and medical conferences. This is a very real problem for those living with cancer because it means that lots of crucial research often fails to reach those who need it the most.

Having taught cancer-specific nutritional courses in a wide variety of settings over the years, I have consistently found both of these twin issues of complexity and access to be the primary barriers that prevent those living with cancer from adopting a robust and evidence-based dietary framework. Fortunately, there is an incredibly simple, intuitive and time-tested answer to this problem, which is always my first port of call when teaching people how to optimise the anti-cancer potential of their diet, and that's the famous six tastes of Ayurveda. This approach provides us with a clear and all-encompassing roadmap to direct what we should be eating in a way that is comprehensive, evidence-based, simple and sustainable. To note that in keeping with the simplicity of the six tastes concept, although herbs and spices are different in botanical terms, they are both considered as herbs in the sphere of Ayurvedic herbal medicines. Therefore, you will find that spices like ginger and turmeric are often described as herbs in this context, as is the case in this book too.

However, before we explore this framework in detail, we need to step back and contextualise how, and in what ways, nutritional medicine can be of actual specific value and relevance to cancer survivorship. When we read about 'cancer-fighting foods' or 'anti-cancer foods', what do we actually mean? What are the quantifiable and evidence-based mechanisms through which food can directly interact with and inhibit cancer cell biology? Exploring such questions is important because it provides validity around the merit of modifying our diet when living with cancer. It is also incredibly motivating. When we know, as just one example, that ginger contains a plethora of phytocompounds that have been reliably shown to induce programmed cell death in cancer cells, it is much more likely that we will be motivated to drink ginger tea on a daily basis. Why? Because we have faith in the validity of the science behind doing so. Expand this singular example across all the evidence in all the primary food groups and suddenly the confusion, frustration and overwhelm that so often clouds our decisions around how best to optimise our diet in the face of cancer is replaced with a genuine sense of clarity and empowerment. If we are to explore this topic in a meaningful way, it is imperative that our starting point is understanding the very foundational hallmarks of cancer and how to suppress them.

## The Hallmarks of Cancer and Anti-Cancer Nutrition

It should come as no surprise that the vegetable kingdom in the broadest sense is the richest natural source of chemo-preventative (that is to say, cancer preventing and destroying) agents. This is a fact best highlighted by the sheer number of conventional anti-cancer drugs that originate from plant compounds. Consider this: across all the anti-cancer pharmaceutical drugs licensed from 1940 to 2002, 69 per cent of these were developed from compounds derived exclusively from plants.[2] This is a staggering statistic and one that highlights in a very significant way the perhaps unparalleled cancer-managing potential to be found in the natural world. And in a practical sense, our diet is the simplest and most powerful way of harnessing this potential and unleashing it in our own bodies. But to do so in a scientifically valid way, there are two questions that we have to ask of the current body of cancer-specific nutritional research:

1. Is there a systematic and comprehensive understanding of the primary mechanisms that cancer cells use to fuel their development, progression and spread?
2. If so, is there scientifically robust and clinically reliable evidence to show that dietary compounds can effectively inhibit and suppress such mechanisms?

With these two foundational questions answered, we would then be in a position to understand clearly the specific foods we need to be consuming on a daily basis and how to build a framework of adoption around these foods. Fortunately, research over the last several decades has provided near unequivocal answers to these two questions. More specifically, the pioneering work of professors Douglas Hanahan and Robert Weinberg has been instrumental in creating clinical consensus around the primary physiological, immunological and metabolic mechanisms employed by cancer cells that allows them to fuel growth, evade immune destruction and invade distant parts of the body. They labelled this framework 'the hallmarks of cancer', which to date represents the gold standard in understanding the interdependent and multifactorial mechanisms of cancer promotion.[3] Through cultivating a clearer understanding of the multifactorial mechanisms that cancer uses to ensure its survival and promotion in this way, it has guided and informed a clearer understanding of how to develop treatments and approaches to counter these mechanisms in new and novel ways.

One such novel approach is via the application of nutritional medicine and the study of how different foods, and the unique phytonutrients they contain, are able to reliably and evidentially suppress these primary hallmarks of cancer promotion. The overarching conclusion that can be drawn from this evidence, which spans decades of research across thousands of publications, is that there are a whole raft of foods and specific phytonutrients that are able to evidentially suppress *all* the hallmarks of cancer promotion identified and documented by Hanahan and Weinberg. Thus, in response to our two questions, we can be absolutely clear that there is both a clear understanding of the primary mechanisms used by cancer cells to promote their survival and progression, and an equally clear understanding of how nutritional medicine can be used to help suppress such mechanisms. It is, therefore, no longer a question of can nutritional intervention positively and evidentially be used as a supportive therapy in cancer care but rather what foods are most effective in their capacity to do so and which specific hallmarks of cancer do they proactively address. To answer this, it is important for us to explore exactly what these hallmarks of cancer are and how food can be used to inhibit them.

## Suppression of Cancer Hallmark 1: Inducing Cancer Cell Apoptosis

All healthy cells in the body contain an encoded message that regulates their lifespan. When any given healthy cell reaches the end of its lifespan, or if the cell becomes damaged, a process called apoptosis is initiated by specific enzymes found within the cell. This causes the cell to die so that it can be replaced by a healthy new cell. In such a way, the dynamic regeneration of the body continues as old makes way for new. Unfortunately, however, cancerous cells employ a variety of mechanisms that allow them to either evade or deactivate this form of programmed cell death. It is this ability to evade apoptosis that allows for the dangerous and unregulated proliferation of cellular growth that we know to be the hallmark of cancer. Reactivating apoptosis in cancer cells is one of the key clinical targets in the development of new and novel anti-cancer drugs.[4] Similarly, the last twenty years has also seen an explosion of clinical research into the testing of myriad nutritional compounds relevant to their ability to induce apoptosis in cancer cells.[5] And what this research now shows it that there are a wide variety of foods, such as kale, extra-virgin olive oil, shiitake mushrooms and certain stone fruit, that are clinically proven to stimulate apoptosis in cancer cells in this way. We will explore such foods in detail later in this chapter.

## Suppression of Cancer Hallmark 2: Inhibiting Angiogenesis

The next hallmark of cancer suppression that is absolutely vital to address via nutritional intervention is the inhibition of a physiological process called angiogenesis. When a cancer first starts to grow, it can only grow to a certain size before a higher volume of oxygen and nutrient-rich blood is needed to fuel subsequent growth. To facilitate this, cancer cells release a chemical called angiogenin, which attracts or 'forces' new blood vessels to grow towards the tumour and then attach to it. This allows it to access a much larger supply of nutrients, which in turn facilitates a quicker rate of cell proliferation and growth. This process is called angiogenesis (*angio* being Greek for 'vessel' and *genesis* meaning 'new birth'). If growth continues, cancerous cells can often begin the process of invading neighbouring tissue to set up distant satellite sites throughout the body, a process called metastasis.

However, satellite cancer sites such as these typically die off very quickly unless they can develop a new supply of blood vessels to sustain them. To do this, they again initiate the process of angiogenesis. Fortunately, there is a counterbalance to this process in the form of a compound called angiostatin that is able to inhibit the ability of cancer cells to pull in the new blood vessels they need to fuel growth. In the absence of a new fuel supply, cancer cells are very much forced into submission. Today, there are a host of pharmaceutical anti-cancer drugs, such as Avastin, which work on preventing angiogenesis in this way. However, there are also a wide selection of robustly trialled nutritional compounds that have been shown to inhibit the process of angiogenesis, including certain types of mushrooms, green tea, turmeric and garlic.[6] As such, the widespread integration of angiogenesis-inhibiting foods is an essential component of a robust anti-cancer diet.

## Suppression of Cancer Hallmark 3:
## Cancer-Specific Immune Activation

The capacity of the mammalian immune system to overcome the threat of cancer is truly profound and, in many ways, unparalleled. While the medical and biological sciences have progressed rapidly in their understanding of how the immune system works and responds in the face of cancer, much is still left to be discovered. Such discoveries require a deeper understanding of the often idiosyncratic behaviour and impacts of immune activity relevant to cancer containment and destruction. For example, why it is that in some cases the body is able to mount an immune response of such ferociousness that even advanced cancers have been beaten into full and impossible remission, and yet in other cases the body is unable to unleash such an assault.[7]

These are questions of profound importance because the clinical evidence clearly highlights that immune status and activity specifically within the tumour microenvironment is a significant and reliable predictor of cancer progression rates, prognoses and survival times.[8] And while this is not true of all cancers all the time, it is true for most cancers most of the time and is thus of importance and relevance to us. Fortunately, the health and functionality of our immune system is largely in our own hands, and in this respect nutritional medicine takes centre stage. The vegetable kingdom contains myriad compounds that are clinically proven in their ability to activate and optimise the cancer-targeting activity of our immune cells. Thus our third dietary mechanism revolves around ensuring that we are harnessing these benefits in the most effective way possible.

## Suppression of Cancer Hallmark 4:
## Suppressing Cancer-Mediated Inflammatory Responses

The next anti-cancer hallmark that it is essential for us to specifically and proactively target via our nutritional practices is the suppression of cancer-mediated inflammatory mechanisms. Inflammation is a natural and vital process that the body initiates to repair tissue damage. For instance, if you were to cut yourself on a sharp knife, your body would increase the production of a chemical called platelet-derived growth factor (PDGF), which, through a complex process of events, stimulates the increased growth of cells in the damaged tissue so that the trauma can be repaired more quickly. Once the damaged tissue has been adequately repaired, the signal to stimulate the growth of new cells stops.

This is an incredibly well-calibrated system that ensures cell growth is stimulated when it is needed and restricted when it isn't. However, cancer is able to hijack this inflammatory pathway to relentlessly fuel its own growth. So important is this mechanism that clinical evidence has observed that inflammatory status in those with cancer is one of the most accurate and clinically significant predictors of health status and survival times.[9] Of particular relevance in this context is the role played by one of the most sinister and destructive tools that cancer cells use to fuel growth, an inflammatory compound called nuclear factor-kappa B (NF-κB). Virtually every action that cancer cells use to promote their own survival is supported by the role of NF-κB.[10] Consequently, the suppression of cancer-mediated inflammatory activity is of utmost importance. Fortunately, there is an abundance of clinical research relevant to cancer cell biology on the ability of a whole host of fruits, vegetables, herbs and spices to inhibit this process, as we shall explore in detail later in this chapter.

## Suppression of Cancer Hallmark 5: Evading Growth Inhibitors

A defining clinical characteristic of a cancer cell is its ability to evade the natural cell cycle suppressors that govern healthy cell replication. While there are many mechanisms in the body that are responsible for regulating healthy cell replication in this way, it is the unique actions of the p53 gene that reign supreme. Clinical evidence now shows that it is very difficult for a healthy cell to become cancerous unless the activity of the p53 gene is deactivated.[11]

The cancer-suppressing activity of p53 is so significant that it is colloquially known as the 'guardian of the genome'. However, the majority of cancers have developed advanced mechanisms to evade p53 genetic suppression. This is best observed by the fact that p53 mutation occurs in well over 50 per cent of all human cancers. When the p53 gene becomes mutant in this way, it is no longer able to control and inhibit cell replication rates, thereby allowing cancer cell growth to progress in an unrestricted way. Furthermore, p53 gene mutations play a key role in promoting cancer cells' ability to invade neighbouring tissue, support metastasis and acquire a greater resistance against conventional cancer treatments such as chemotherapy. As a result, the reactivation of the genetic cancer-suppressing mechanisms such as p53 is important. There is now growing consensus around the ability of nutritional compounds to help facilitate this, particularly in the form of the phytonutrients found in foods such as berries, tomatoes and cruciferous vegetables.

## Suppression of Cancer Hallmark 6: Suppressing Proliferative Growth Signalling

The aggressive and uncontrolled proliferation of cell division has been described as 'the most fundamental trait of cancer cells'. To support this proliferation, cancer cells display a significantly increased response to cell growth stimulants alongside increased impunity from the physiological controls that are responsible for the tight regulation of such mechanisms. This allows cancerous cells to proliferate at dangerous speeds to dangerous levels. Research shows that dietary variables are a 'major influencer affecting growth factor levels as well as other aspects related to cancer cell proliferation and can influence the onset and development of cancers in a variety of different ways'.[12] In particular, foods such as celery, chamomile tea, parsley and omega-3 fatty acids have all be shown to suppress a selection of key cell proliferative pathways in this way.

## Suppression of Cancer Hallmark 7: Inhibiting the Mechanisms of Metastases

Our seventh and final hallmark focuses on the suppression of the mechanisms that cancers use to metastasise to distant parts of the body. This is fundamentally important because the life-threatening potential of cancer is often misunderstood and misrepresented. Localised or contained cancers are rarely life threatening. It is only when cancers migrate to distant parts of the body and establish colonies there that they truly become dangerous. Indeed, over 80 per cent of all cancer deaths are caused by metastasised cancers.[13] Intervening in a way that can help to suppress the mechanisms that cancer cells use to metastasise is thus of vital importance. Currently, a growing foundation of evidence is highlighting the importance of a variety of nutritional compounds in this capacity. For example, the celebrated phytonutrient epigallocatechin-3-gallate (EGCG), found in green tea, and the curcumin found in turmeric have been shown to inhibit a variety of the physiological mechanisms that cancer cells use to promote metastatic growth and invasion.[14]

## The Practical Application of Suppressing the Seven Hallmarks of Cancer

When adopting an evidence-based anti-cancer diet, the priority is to ensure we are consuming foods that target *all seven* of these primary hallmarks of cancer suppression each and every day. The best way to achieve this is to increase the breadth and variety of the anti-cancer foods we consume.

Perhaps the best way of articulating the fundamental importance of nutritional breadth is via the analogy of the home security system. Imagine you wanted to instal the most advanced home security system due to a spate of house burglaries in your neighbourhood. It uses the best sensors, locks and monitors, and you feel your home is impregnable. Which it is. And yet despite the unquestionable robustness of the security system you have adopted, imagine one day before leaving home you accidentally forget to shut the fanlight window in your bathroom. This one small and relatively insignificant oversight is ultimately enough to compromise the security of your entire home and allow a burglar to break in, despite all the measures you have taken to defend it.

So, too, with our diet. A robust anti-cancer diet only truly becomes so if we are successfully targeting all seven of these hallmarks of cancer suppression on a daily basis. Successfully targeting six of these hallmarks while failing to address the seventh is akin to us leaving the bathroom window open; the integrity of the entire system is compromised. Thus, what is needed is a clear and simple framework for ensuring the daily addition of foods that target all of these hallmarks; here, the concept of the six tastes of Ayurveda represents arguably the most holistic and intuitive way of doing so.

## The Six Tastes of Ayurveda as an Anti-Cancer Nutritional Blueprint

The founding fathers of Ayurveda intuitively understood the central importance of nutrition in the quest for optimal health and disease management. Realising this importance, it become imperative to them that a clear, systematic and tailored approach to nutritional medicine was created. This was a model that needed to ensure the provision of enough dietary breadth and variety to unleash the full healing capacity of nutritional medicine but in a way that was simple to understand and easy to implement. The framework that was subsequently developed, tested and refined to fulfil these nutritional goals was the now revered six tastes of Ayurveda, which represents one of the most beautifully unique and comprehensive approaches to nutrition ever developed.

In this model, all foods can be classified as belonging to one or more of the six primary tastes: sweet, salty, sour, bitter, pungent and astringent. Ironically, however, the first thing to emphasise about these six tastes is that they are less a way of classifying how foods taste in the mouth and more a way of classifying the impact they have upon the chemical, enzymatic and physiological workings of the body. For instance, some foods clearly match the taste they belong to – salt tastes salty and lemons taste sour. But such examples across the length and breadth of the food we eat are rare.

What is of more relevance and importance to us is the way different foods, and the unique nutrients, chemicals and compounds they contain, go on to modulate the physiological workings of the body upon being eaten and digested. For example, if you were to peel a thumbnail-sized piece of fresh ginger, pop it into your mouth and chew it, what would be the response? The intensely pungent compounds found within ginger, such as zingiberene and gingerol, would immediately increase saliva production and the sensation of heat in the mouth. It would also vasodilate the capillaries in our mouth and face. And once swallowed, it would increase hydrochloric acid production in our stomach and through doing so have a direct impact upon speeding up and strengthening our digestive capacity. Thus, when we say ginger is a pungent food, we are less interested in our subjective interpretation of the taste in our mouth and more interested in the objective way it goes on to regulate and modify the physiological workings of the body.

This is the central concept of the six tastes of Ayurveda and one that can be extrapolated across to the actions of all foods, including their specific anti-cancer actions. Some of the most important anti-cancer foods are those found within the bitter taste, and kale is one such food. Kale contains myriad phytochemicals such as sulforaphane, which is responsible, in part, for its strong bitter flavour. However, sulforaphane is also a powerful and proven anti-cancer compound that targets several of the hallmarks of cancer suppression, such as inhibiting angiogenesis and promoting apoptosis.[15] So while kale does taste bitter, it is the chemicals that make up this bitterness, and the anti-cancer mechanisms they modulate, that are of most relevance to us. But the beauty of this way of eating is that almost all vegetables from within the bitter taste (and many from the sweet taste) also contain sulforaphane. So, by ensuring the daily intake of foods across the bitter taste, we can be confident that we are supporting the body with the proven anti-cancer compounds they contain in a simple and sustainable way by focusing on the overarching taste, in this case bitter, rather than fixating on any specific individual food.

This viewpoint holds true for all the other six tastes too and the unique anti-cancer compounds they contain. And this is why the six tastes of Ayurveda are so important; they act as a profoundly effective and all-encompassing roadmap for guiding us on what to eat in a way that unlocks all of the benefits of cancer-specific nutrition in a simple, easy and sustainable way. So, let us explore exactly what these six tastes are, the foods they contain and the anti-cancer activity inherent within them.

## Taste 1: Anabolic (classically labelled 'sweet')

Before launching into an exploration of this taste, a small caveat: in classical Ayurveda and almost every other Ayurvedic textbook you will read, this taste is called 'sweet'. In this book, I would like to break away from that label and instead classify these foods as 'anabolic'. Anabolic foods are those that have a strengthening, building and physiologically rejuvenating impact upon the body. The reason I would like to alter the title of this taste from sweet to anabolic is that cancer is a largely metabolic disease and the majority of cancers need glucose, and lots of it, to fuel growth. This is why reducing our consumption of refined sugars and white carbohydrates is of such importance. By labelling this taste as sweet there is a risk of: 1) scaring people into thinking that Ayurveda advocates the daily adoption of unhealthy, high-sugar foods (which it doesn't); or 2) suggesting that eating these kinds of refined, high-glucose foods is acceptable as part of an evidence-based anti-cancer diet (which it isn't). The labelling of these foods as anabolic circumvents this issue while still being true to the wonderfully energising and strengthening impact they have upon the body and the wealth of nutrient-dense anti-cancer foods and nutrients they contain, the most important of which are explored below,

## The Primary Anabolic Foods and Their Anti-Cancer Actions
### CAROTENOID-RICH FRUITS AND VEGETABLES
Root vegetables such as carrots, beetroot and sweet potatoes, along with squashes and pumpkins, are anti-cancer powerhouses, primarily due to the high levels of carotenoids they contain, such as beta-carotenoids, alpha carotenoids and lutein. A large foundation of evidence exists to highlight the ability of these phytonutrients to suppress a wide variety of cancer cells.[16] The focus of this research largely centres on the relationship between carotenoids and a specific protein called C43.

All healthy cells have C43 proteins on their surfaces. When these proteins come into contact with other healthy cells also possessing C43 proteins, it directly controls and regulates the growth and replication of the cells in a process called 'cell contact inhibition'. Cancer cells have very few C43 proteins on their surface, which in part explains their ability to continue to proliferate in a more uncontrolled and aggressive way. Research shows that carotenoids are able to stimulate C43 activity in cancer cells in a way that encourages them to revert to normal cellular behaviour.[17] This may explain the consistently observed anti-proliferative impacts of high-carotenoid foods. The phytonutrient composition of high-carotenoid fruits and vegetables also plays an important role in cancer-specific immune and inflammatory modulation. A longitudinal study showed that over a six-year trial period, a diet high in carotenoids resulted in a significant extension of survival times in women living with breast cancer.[18]

**To Use:** Add root vegetables widely into curries, stews and casseroles. Fresh beetroot can be used to make anti-cancer beetroot hummus. Finely grate fresh carrots and beetroots into salads and sandwiches. All these vegetables are excellent roasted and can be added to warm or cold salads and as healthier additions to roast dinners.

## EXTRA-VIRGIN OLIVE OIL

One of the most valuable health-promoting and disease-suppressing foods in the world, extra-virgin olive oil is a central component of an inclusive anti-cancer diet. While also possessing a level of pungency, healthy oils such as extra-virgin olive oil are primarily classified as being an anabolic food. Crucially, extra-virgin olive oil contains oleocanthal, a potent anti-cancer antioxidant. Oleocanthal is made when olives are crushed to make the oil. Evidence shows that oleocanthal is able to puncture and invade cancer cell lysosomes, which are where cells dispose of waste. Although lysosomes are found in most animal cells, cancer cells often have larger and more numerous lysosomes, making them more vulnerable to oleocanthal attack than other cells. Clinical studies have now shown that via the targeting of the lysosomes in this way, oleocanthal is able to induce apoptosis, or cell death, in a variety of cancers, including breast, pancreatic and prostate cancer cells.[19] Similarly, oleocanthal has been shown to suppress breast and prostate cancer cell proliferation and inhibit their ability to invade and metastasise to distant parts of the body while also supporting immune-mediated cancer cell destruction.[20] And because the majority of the myriad anti-cancer compounds found in extra-virgin olive oil are fat soluble, meaning they are absorbed into fatty tissue, they have a particular affinity for the inhibition of tumours forming in fatty tissue, such as breast and uterine cancers.

**To Use:** Drizzle widely over salads, soups and most savoury dishes. Use in dips and as an alternative to butter on breads, and to make herbal marinades for fish, vegetables and meats. The suggested dose is around two tablespoons a day.

## GHEE

Ghee is a form of clarified butter that is made by gently heating unsalted butter until the milk solids separate from the fat. The melted butter is then strained to remove all the milk solids, leaving pure butter fat, which is the ghee. It is one of the most revered foods in the Ayurvedic framework and comes with a vast array of health benefits. Crucially, ghee is one of the highest natural sources of conjugated linoleic acid, which in clinical studies has been shown to induce cell death in human cancer cells.[21] Moreover, conjugated linoleic acid has also been shown to possess important immunostimulatory properties, specifically relevant to the activity of a type of immune cell called

T-cells, which play a central role in the effective identification and destruction of cancer cells.[22] Ghee is arguably the highest source of butyric acid, a short-chain fatty acid, which is essential for the proper functioning of the human microbiome found within the gut. Not only is the health of the microbiome directly responsible for up to 70 per cent of our collective immune activity but in clinical studies butyric acid has been shown to suppress proliferative signalling in certain types of cancer, thereby inhibiting their growth cycle.[23]

**To Use:** Ghee can be easily adopted into your daily diet by using it as your first-choice oil whenever frying anything in a pan or simply by melting a teaspoon or two into porridge, soups, stews or curries. Another great way of using ghee is in the famous Ojas Tonic recipe. You can find this in the Recipes and Meal Plan section of this book's online resources, at www.mind-body-medical.co.uk/becomingexceptional.

### SWEET STONE FRUITS

In the Ayurvedic tradition, sweet, ripe stones fruits, such as plums, nectarines and peaches, are revered for the nourishing and rejuvenating impact they have upon human physiology. This is a view strongly replicated in the clinical anti-cancer research, which shows these kinds of stone fruits to possess efficacy in suppressing many of the hallmarks of cancer previously discussed. For example, two of the anti-cancer phytonutrients found in these types of fruit – phenolic compounds and anthocyanins – have been shown to inhibit the process cancer cells use to evade apoptosis while at the same time stimulating cancer cell death.[24] These phytonutrients have also been shown to reduce proliferative signalling among a wide variety of cancer cells while also reducing their ability to invade neighbouring tissue.[25]

**To Use:** Try to eat one to two stone fruits a day as a healthy anti-cancer snack between meals. Stone fruits are also fantastic when gently stewed; add some chopped dates, nuts and seeds, a little cinnamon and some melted ghee for a quick and tasty anti-cancer breakfast.

### WHOLEGRAINS

The integration of unprocessed and unrefined complex carbohydrates into an authentic anti-cancer diet, in moderation, is important. Such foods provide energy and vitality to the body in a simple and easy-to-assimilate format. Furthermore, epidemiological research now links the regular intake of wholegrains to a reduced risk of cancer occurrence and reoccurrence.[26] These benefits are believed to be due to the potent phytonutrient make-up of wholegrains, such as phenolic acids, carotenoids, alkylresorcinols, phytosterols, lignans, anthocyanins, vitamin E and polysaccharides. Several studies show that wholegrains exert powerful anti-cancer activity via the suppression of several of the hallmarks of cancer, including the suppression of cell proliferation, modulating anti-cancer immune activity, supporting apoptosis and suppressing metastatic growth, particularly in breast cancer cells.[27]

**To Use:** Great options for harnessing these benefits include grains such as spelt, millet, rye, barley, sorghum and oats. However, a word of caution: in most cases, shop-bought breads and products using wholegrains will contain excess sugar and damaging ultra-processed compounds such as emulsifiers. When looking for pure wholegrain products, check the ingredient list to ensure it contains only natural ingredients that you recognise. Alternatively, invest in a bread maker, buy organic wholegrain flours and make your own homemade bread, which you can enjoy in the absence of any nasty chemicals, toxins or additives.

### NUTS AND SEEDS

Nut and seeds are among the most nutritionally dense foods in the world and ones that are consistently linked to better health profiles in large population studies. One of the key reasons for this is the presence of the celebrated omega-3 fatty acids found in nuts and seeds. Not only are omega-3 fatty acids vital for supporting optimal brain and heart health but they also possess anti-cancer properties. The vegetal omega-3 fatty acids found in nuts and seeds have powerful immune-modulating and anti-inflammatory impacts relevant to cancer.[28] However, perhaps one of the most important anti-cancer mechanisms attributed to omega-3 is its ability to suppress NF-κB. As explored in Suppressing Cancer-Mediated Inflammatory Responses on page 68, NF-κB is implicated in virtually every action that cancer cells use to fuel growth and promote their own survival. Research shows that the nutritional compounds found within omega-3 can help to neutralise the actions of NF-κB in a powerful way. This explains, in part, the epidemiological data highlighting why those eating a diet high in omega-3 have a lower incidence of cancer.[29]

**To Use:** Nuts such as almonds, cashews, macadamia nuts, walnuts and Brazil nuts, alongside seeds such as hemp and flax, are ideal ways of adding more omega-3 into your diet. These can be snacked on when hungry, ground up and added to smoothies or porridge, or lightly toasted and mixed into salads.

**OTHER IMPORTANT ANABOLIC FOODS**
In addition to the specific anti-cancer foods discussed, this taste also includes a selection of other foods that we should widely include within our diets, such as: avocados, sweet apples, mangoes, coconut, prunes, dates, figs, oats, wholegrain/wholewheat rice, pastas and breads (in moderation), organic grass-fed meat and wild-caught fish (if you are eating animal products) and raw honey for when a little sweetness is required.

## Taste 2: Salty

The salty taste is both the smallest and easiest taste to understand and use. In today's world we are all too familiar with the salty taste as it pervades virtually all processed and ultra-processed foods. And it is undeniable that too much salt, particularly processed table salts that contain dangerously high levels of sodium, is bad for us. Despite this, using the right kind of natural and unprocessed salt in the right way and in the correct dose is vital. Salt is absolutely essential for the proper regulation of many actions and systems of the body; it provides vital minerals, it conducts nerve impulses, regulates muscle activity and maintains the proper balance of water and minerals. Similarly, salt plays an important role in the optimal functioning of the digestive system. And while pure salt doesn't possess any specific anti-cancer actions, we can best think of it as a 'synergising' taste, meaning that its addition allows us to better benefit from all of the powerful anti-cancer properties found in the other five tastes. To harness these benefits, we don't need to do much more than ensure we moderately season our food with salt. However, not all salt it created equal, and if we are using salt daily, it is important to delineate the three most common types of salt available.

**Common Table Salt:** This is to be avoided at all costs. It is highly processed to increase its sodium content, which makes it more damaging to the body. Table salt also contains lots of additives that are used in the refining process, primarily aluminium.

**Sea Salt:** This is one of the purest types of salt and simply involves drying sea water in the sun to produce salt crystals. Sea salt has an excellent mineral profile and imparts a lovely taste in cooking. However, it is essential to only use naturally dried sea salt rather than desalinated sea salt as the latter uses lots of chemicals that are damaging to the health of the body.

**Mineral Salt:** This type of salt has shot to fame over the last decade with the increased knowledge of pink Himalayan salt. Mineral salt is harvested from ancient sea beds that dried up many millennia ago. Mineral salt is a fantastic product because it contains hard-to-obtain trace minerals, such as calcium, magnesium, potassium, copper and iron, all of which are essential to the proper functioning of the body. It also contains only around 85 per cent sodium compared to table salt, which is over 99 per cent sodium. For this reason, mineral salt such as pink Himalayan salt is my preferred option.

However, while salt in its pure form doesn't possess any specific or isolated anti-cancer benefits, there is one classification of food from within the salty taste that does and that's sea vegetables such as seaweed. A growing foundation of evidence highlights the ability of certain types of seaweed, such as nori, dulse and kombu/kelp, to slow down the proliferation rates of many different types of cancer.[30] Furthermore, edible seaweeds are powerful immune stimulants that have been shown to specifically increase the number of circulating natural killer cells, which are among the most important immune cells relevant to cancer suppression.

**To Use:** Dried seaweeds and seaweed flakes are readily available at most big supermarkets or online and these can be readily added to casseroles and soups. You can even buy sea spaghetti to use in Italian dishes.

## Taste 3: Sour

The sour taste is a therapeutically important but often overlooked one in the Western world. It is also a taste that contains a core selection of powerful anti-cancer foods that need to be integrated into our daily diet, so it should not be neglected. In terms of the actual taste, sour foods are those that, to varying degrees, induce the type of lip-puckering response we experience if we were to bite into a fresh lemon. Most natural and unprocessed sour foods are incredibly nutrient dense and contain a wide variety of phytonutrients that possess proven immune-supporting, health-promoting and anti-cancer actions. Interestingly, in the primary European longevity zones – areas of the world with the highest percentage of healthy and independent centenarians – lemon and limes are used extensively in most meals, including the zest, juice and actual fruit. Current thinking suggests that the subtle but continual use of sour foods in this way helps to support optimal digestion, enhanced gut-based immunity and inflammation modulation while also providing lots of vitamin C and other key antioxidants. These are foods that we want to be benefiting from on a daily basis.

## The Primary Sour Foods and Their Anti-Cancer Actions
### CITRUS FRUITS

Fruits such as lemons, limes, oranges and grapefruits are immensely high in a wide variety of phytonutrients, such as vitamins B and C, and essential minerals, such as potassium, phosphorous, magnesium and copper. Citrus fruits also house over sixty different varieties of flavonoids[31] and it is these that are largely responsible for the potent anti-cancer actions they possess. Current evidence highlights that these dietary flavonoids interfere with carcinogen activation, stimulate carcinogen detoxification, scavenge free radicals, control cell-cycle progression, induce apoptosis, inhibit cell proliferation, suppress angiogenesis and help to block the mechanisms cancer cells use to invade distant parts of the body.[32]

**To Use:** Drizzle fresh lemon juice over your meals, make marinades from the juice, make fresh lemon and ginger tea and grate lemon and lime peel over salads (be sure to use organic fruits if doing this).

### BERRIES

Berries such as blueberries, raspberries, gooseberries, blackberries and strawberries are among the most nutritionally dense fruits in the world. Ayurvedically speaking, these types of berries straddle the anabolic (sweet) and sour tastes, but the latter typically predominates. These fruits are well researched within the field of anti-cancer nutrition and have consistently been shown to possess powerful cancer-suppressing actions. Specifically, studies have reported beneficial effects of berries or their constituents on the modulation of inflammation, the inhibition of angiogenesis, the stimulation of apoptosis and the inhibition of cancer cell proliferation rates.[33]

**To Use:** Arguably the best and simplest way to harness the benefits of berries is to use them as an anti-cancer snack between meals, aiming to eat a handful of berries each day. Frozen berries are an excellent way to use berries out of season and these can be mixed into porridge or added to smoothies. Of course, in the summer, try growing your own organic berries, and don't forget to get foraging for fresh blackberries in early autumn; these can be frozen to see you through winter. Not only does this provide us with a free supply of anti-cancer superfoods but it also comes with the added benefit of getting us outside and engaged with the natural world, which is a healing entity in and of itself.

### TOMATOES

Ayurvedically speaking, tomatoes pose a slight problem as they are not advocated due to the very stimulating effects they have on the body and mind. However, in light of the proven anti-cancer benefits they possess, I think it is justified to include them here with a small caveat: tomatoes are best eaten when fully ripe, well cooked and ideally in season. The proven anti-cancer benefits of tomatoes are primarily attributed to the high levels of lycopene they contain. Lycopene is a specific type of carotenoid that gives tomatoes their bright red colour. Clinical research has observed that lycopene's anti-cancer impacts are due to its ability to interfere with cancer cell migration mechanisms, inhibit invasion into neighbouring tissue, suppress angiogenesis and promote apoptosis.[34]

**To Use:** It is important to emphasise that the bioavailability of lycopene is greatly enhanced by cooking. Thus, try making your own Italian pasta sauces using fresh tomatoes. Also, fried tomatoes on wholegrain toast drizzled with olive oil and served with some quickly fried kale and garlic is a great breakfast option.

### PROBIOTIC FOODS

The clinical interest around the use and impact of probiotics has exploded in recent years, and for good reason; it is impossible to live in a healthy body without a healthy gut for the simple fact that the gut microbiome, and the trillions of healthy bacteria and other microbes found within it, informs the very foundation upon which the optimal physiological workings of the body are built. This is particularly true of the immune system, over 70 per cent of which is produced within the gut. Furthermore, new research shows that the gut microbiota is able to orchestrate a variety of cancer-specific immune alterations that allow certain immune cells, such as natural killer cells, to better identify and destroy cancer cells.[35]

Supporting a healthy gut is, therefore, imperative. And while we will be exploring this topic in more detail in the following chapter, it is worth highlighting here the role played by certain probiotic and fermented foods that belong to the sour taste. Chief among these are foods such as sauerkraut, apple cider vinegar, live yogurt and kefir. All these foods contain concentrated strains of healthy bacteria that help to continually support and repopulate the bacterial growth within the microbiota. The adoption of these kinds of probiotic foods into our daily diet is an important addition, both in the context of general health optimisation and also the specific anti-cancer mechanisms they support.

**To Use:** While there are instances in which specific probiotic supplements are clinically indicated (such as after antibiotic treatment), generally speaking we can obtain enough probiotic support from our diet. Try to ensure your weekly shop contains a variety of probiotic foods, such as sauerkraut, apple cider vinegar, live yogurt and kefir, and simply adopt these into your daily diet in a way that best suits you.

**OTHER IMPORTANT SOUR FOODS**
Grapefruit, kiwi fruit, sheep and goat's cheese (in moderation).

## Taste 4: Bitter

The bitter taste includes some of the most health- and longevity-promoting foods in the world, chief among these being dark leafy green vegetables, such as kale, chard, dandelions, spring and winter greens, and pak choi. This taste also includes most of the cruciferous vegetables, such as broccoli and cabbage, healthy treats such as dark chocolate, and also coffee. Unfortunately, the bitter taste is becoming increasingly absent from the standard Western diet as the increased exposure to refined sugars is making it more and more unpalatable. However, it is vital to mobilise the anti-cancer actions inherent within healthy bitter foods in our daily diets and the recipes found in the online Recipes and Meal Plan lean heavily into the use of bitter foods (see www.mind-body-medical.co.uk/becomingexceptional).

## The Primary Bitter Foods and Their Anti-Cancer Actions
### LEAFY GREEN VEGETABLES AND CRUCIFERS

Leafy green vegetables, such as kale, spinach, collard greens, Swiss chard, greens and pak choi, and other crucifers, such as broccoli, cabbage and sprouts, are among the most nutritionally dense anti-cancer foods yet identified. This is largely due to the high volumes of anti-cancer phytochemicals such sulforaphane, isothiocyanates and indoles (such as the celebrated indo-3-carbinoles) found within these bitter foods. Clinical research has observed that these powerful plant-based compounds are able to suppress cancer-mediated inflammatory mechanisms, activate cancer-suppressor genes, promote apoptosis in a wide variety of cancer cells, slow proliferation rates and reduce tissue invasion.[36] Laboratory studies have observed that rats possessing high levels of sulforaphane were more than 50 per cent less likely to develop metastases as those rats with low levels.[37]

**To Use:** Boiling these types of vegetables destroys a large percentage of the anti-cancer compounds found within them. The best way to cook them is to very quickly steam or stir-fry them in hot ghee or coconut oil for a few minutes until al dente. Try to add a serving of leafy greens to at least one meal a day. Broccoli and cabbage can be finely grated and added raw to salads.

### COFFEE

In the Ayurvedic tradition, it is viewed as being important to moderate coffee consumption because of the stimulatory impact it can have upon the nervous system. This is particularly true if you suffer with ailments such as anxiety, poor sleep, restlessness and stress. However, in moderation and drunk only in the first half of the day, coffee possesses clear and proven anti-cancer actions. It has long been observed in public health research that coffee consumption is inversely related to cancer risk. And over the last decade, much research has aimed to unpick the mechanisms responsible for this. What this has revealed is that coffee is one of the most phytonutrient-dense foods in the world, containing well over one thousand individual plant-based compounds. When analysed, many of these compounds have been shown to activate a variety of cancer-suppressing mechanisms including the ability to prevent cell proliferation, induce apoptosis, activate cancer-specific immune responses and suppress tumour angiogenesis.[38] Given the validity of this research, enjoying one to two cups of organic coffee a day, ideally before lunchtime, affords a real hit of anti-cancer benefits. If you don't drink coffee, this by no means suggests you should start. But if you do enjoy the taste and ritual of a mindfully consumed cup of coffee, doing so very much falls within the evidence-based arena of a robust anti-cancer diet.

### DARK CHOCOLATE

This is a food that almost everyone is pleased to see on the list! While processed milk chocolate is universally damaging, dark chocolate made with at least 70 per cent to 80 per cent cocoa is a true superfood. The cocoa bean possesses incredibly high levels of essential anti-cancer compounds, primarily a broad range of polyphenols along with high flavonoid levels. Crucially, researchers have observed that these phytocompounds demonstrate potential to suppress cancer-mediated inflammatory actions and cancer cell proliferation pathways, and also to induce apoptosis in established cancer cells.[39]

**To Use:** Most dark chocolate bars still contain a degree of sugar, so moderation is key here. However, to satisfy a sweet craving, they are a great option and one that contains proven anti-cancer compounds. An even better choice is to buy pure cacao powder as this possesses all of the benefits without the addition of any added sugar. This can be sprinkled into porridge, added to smoothies and used in baking to make healthy anti-cancer treats. Caution: due to the high levels of agricultural toxins found in cacao, it is best to only use organic if possible.

### OTHER IMPORTANT BITTER FOODS
Courgettes, aubergines, asparagus.

## Taste 5: Pungent

The pungent taste is made up of a relatively small group of foods and we only need a little of these. They are very much like the salty and sour foods in that they are complements to a meal rather than the centrepiece. That said, the pungent taste contains a selection of powerful anti-cancer foods that we should integrate into our diet. And while the alliums, such as garlic, onions and leeks, are best reserved for cooking, pungent herbs such as ginger lend themselves perfectly to use in herbal teas, which are a great addition to the anti-cancer dietary framework.

## The Primary Pungent Foods and Their Anti-Cancer Actions

### ALLIUMS

Pungent vegetables like garlic, onions, leeks, shallots and spring onions all contain high concentrations of sulphur compounds such as S-allylmercaptocysteine, diallyl disulfide and S-trityl-L-cysteine. Research shows that these sulphur compounds are able to promote apoptosis and mobilise anti-cancer immune activity against a raft of different cancer cells.[40] Furthermore, the sulphur compounds found in these foods has been shown to help suppress the activity of NF-κB (see Suppressing Cancer-Mediated Inflammatory Responses on page 68). Research has shown that these sulphur compounds can counteract the actions of NF-κB, which may underpin the data highlighting why people who have high-garlic diets have a lower incidence of cancer.[41]

To Use: Increasing your intake of alliums is relatively easy as they greatly enhance the flavour of virtually all meals. Aim to integrate lots of garlic and onions into all your meals and recipes, and add leeks and shallots to stews, casseroles and roasts. Note that the sulphur compounds found in garlic are more actively released and become more bioavailable when the garlic is crushed or finely chopped and left for a little while before cooking. A word of caution: if you suffer with any kind of inflammatory bowel disease, such as ulcerative colitis, diverticulitis or even heartburn, please use these types of pungent foods in moderation due to their inherently heating energy.

### BLACK PEPPER

Black pepper is a true nutritional superfood and one that possesses a disproportionately high volume of unique phytochemicals. In Ayurvedic medicine, black pepper is prized as a synergising herb that enhances the absorption of other nutrients it is combined with. Clinical evidence now supports this notion, showing that the addition of black pepper into a meal significantly increases the volume of vitamins, minerals and other nutrients absorbed.[42] Black pepper also possesses powerful anti-cancer actions. Specifically, the piperine found in black pepper has been shown to suppress cancer stem cell renewal, inhibit cancer cell proliferation and induce apoptosis in cancer cells, while also modifying a variety of mechanisms linked to the inhibition of cancer cell invasion and metastases.[43]

**To Use:** Simply ensure that you season your meals well with black pepper when cooking and also add a good pinch of freshly ground black pepper to your finished meal once plated up.

### GINGER

Ginger is revered as one of the most important herbal medicines in Ayurveda. The health benefits of ginger are as profound as they are evidence-based and impact upon multiple body systems, including the cardiovascular, immunological, respiratory, lymphatic and reproductive systems. Ginger possesses powerful anti-cancer actions that are activated by the unique extracts and compounds found within it, such as gingerols, shogaols, zingiberene and zingerone. Evidence suggests that these potent anti-cancer compounds can induce apoptosis, suppress angiogenesis and inhibit the pro-cancer actions of NF-κB while also reducing cancer-mediated inflammatory mechanisms.[44]

**To Use:** Arguably the best way of harnessing the healing properties of ginger is in fresh tea, which is as tasty as it is simple. To make, grate a one- to two-centimetre piece of fresh ginger and place this into a cup before pouring over boiling water. A few peppercorns and a slice of lemon can also be added. Also try to integrate freshly grated ginger widely into your cooking where appropriate.

### OTHER IMPORTANT PUNGENT FOODS

Watercress, rocket, chilli, mustard greens and horseradish.

## Taste 6: Astringent

The astringent taste is arguably the hardest of the six tastes to connect with. The astringent foods and drinks are those that induce a toning, drying and puckering effect in the mouth when we eat them and also across the wider body when we digest them. We can observe this if we were to bite into a green and very unripe banana, or drink a very dry white wine or a strong cup of black tea. The astringent taste contains a selection of crucial anti-cancer foods, some of which are perhaps the most important and well researched in this capacity, namely turmeric and green tea. Astringent foods are often absent from many people's diets, so this is an important one to consciously and proactively target when shopping and preparing meals.

## The Primary Astringent Foods and Their Anti-Cancer Actions
### GREEN TEA
As one of the most famous anti-cancer foods in the world, green tea has been subjected to an extensive array of clinical research. What this research shows is that green tea, and the unique phytocompounds it contains, are able to promote apoptosis and inhibit angiogenesis in a wide variety of cancer cells while also suppressing the ability of cancer cells to invade and metastasise.[45] Most of these benefits are attributed to a specific type of polyphenol called EGCG, which is found in very high concentrations in green tea.

**To Use:** A dose of around 2.5 grams of green tea leaves a day has been shown to be optimal. However, this equates to around six to ten cups per day. If this is too laborious, a great alternative is to use a form of concentrated and powdered green tea called matcha. A single serving of matcha powder, which is typically mixed into a little water or added into smoothies or porridge, typically equates to around twenty to thirty cups of green tea in a single dose, making it more sustainable long term. Matcha can be easily sourced from any good health food shop or bigger supermarkets.

### TURMERIC
The true celebrity of anti-cancer nutrition, turmeric has been a prized herbal medicine in the Ayurvedic tradition for thousands of years. Indeed, this herb is so valuable that it is affectionately known as the 'golden goddess of Ayurveda'. In our in-depth exploration of anti-cancer herbal medicines in chapter 7 we shall visit turmeric once again, but for now suffice to say that the anti-cancer actions of this herb are as evidence-based as they are profound. In a wide variety of studies, turmeric has been shown to reliably induce apoptosis, suppress angiogenesis, reduce cancer cell proliferation rates, inhibit the actions of NF-κB, promote immune modulation, suppress cancer-specific inflammatory pathways and inhibit invasion into neighbouring tissue.[46] While turmeric contains over one hundred unique phytochemicals, most of these specific anti-cancer impacts are attributed to curcumin, the flavonoid that gives turmeric its bright yellow colour.

**To Use:** In some instances, it is indicated to take turmeric in higher and more medicinal doses (please refer to Using These Herbs on page 134 in chapter 7), but in culinary form aim to consume around one to two teaspoons of powdered turmeric a day. Turmeric can be added into porridge and smoothies, stirred into soups, casseroles and stews, added to curries and mixed with fried onions, garlic or other vegetables. Note: for the body to better assimilate the curcumin found in turmeric, it needs to be mixed with black pepper and an oil such as ghee or extra-virgin olive or coconut oil.

### PULSES

Pulses are evidence-based anti-cancer foods that are often overlooked and underused in the context of cancer-specific nutrition. They include chickpeas, all types of lentils and all forms of beans, such as kidney, mung, adzuki, black and butter beans. Aside from their important cancer-suppressing impacts, pulses are also among the foods most clinically linked to enhanced human longevity.[47] In terms of their anti-cancer impacts, pulses have been shown to reduce inflammatory pathways, protect DNA health, reduce cancer cell proliferation, induce apoptosis and inhibit metastatic activation.[48]

**To Use:** The meaty and filling qualities of pulses, which are a fantastic source of plant-based protein, make them a great way of reducing meat intake. They are incredibly versatile and can be added into most common meals; for example, lentils make a great alternative to minced beef or lamb. And, when made properly, hummus is one of the most densely packed anti-cancer options of them all. (See the accompanying online Recipes and Meal Plan at www.mind-body-medical.co.uk/becomingexceptional for a fantastic anti-cancer hummus recipe.)

### MUSHROOMS

The anti-cancer benefits of mushrooms are profound and the addition of a broad variety of mushrooms into our diet should be a key priority when crafting anti-cancer meals. This is because mushrooms are powerful immune stimulants that activate the full spectrum of cancer suppression pathways, including the ability to induce apoptosis, inhibit angiogenesis, increase cancer-specific immune responses, reduce proliferation rates, suppress tissue invasion and much else besides.[49] Great options here include mushrooms such as shiitake, oyster, maitake, lion's mane, cordyceps and chaga, all of which lend themselves perfectly to use in cooking and drinks. However, we don't always need to use these types of exotic or harder-to-come by varieties as the more commonly available white, button and chestnut mushrooms also contain a wealth of anti-cancer nutrients. All these mushrooms can be sourced dried (or in powdered form) and in many cases fresh.

**To Use:** Add dried or fresh mushrooms to soups, curries and stews; fried, they make a great breakfast option, add to stir-fries, or use powdered in smoothies and drinks.

**OTHER IMPORTANT ASTRINGENT FOODS**
Cranberries, pomegranate, quinoa, buckwheat and celery.

## Using the Six Tastes of Ayurveda in Daily Life

The overarching benefit of using the six tastes of Ayurveda as our primary anti-cancer nutritional roadmap is how easy it is to adopt and the nutritional breadth it affords. For a health-promoting diet to work it must be sustainable long term. And to be sustainable long term it must be easy to use. This is why the six tastes of Ayurveda affords us the master key to unlocking full body anti-cancer nutrition: **because all we have to do is ensure that we include foods from all six tastes in every meal that we prepare and eat, each and every day.** If we can do this, and it is easy to do, we will accumulatively expose the body to an exponential volume of powerful anti-cancer compounds that allow us to harness the best available evidence around anti-cancer nutrition.

By including a wide variety of foods from the different six tastes, we also unleash the arguably unparalleled impacts of nutritional synergy. In Ayurveda, this is a concept of utmost importance and is based upon the view that when we combine a variety of healthy foods together, the whole collective nutritional gain obtained is greater than the sum of the individual foods in that meal. Arguably, the simplest example of this is the beautiful nutritional synergy found between turmeric and black pepper. As we have seen, turmeric contains potent anti-cancer actions. So too does black pepper. But when you combine turmeric with black pepper, the bioavailability of these anti-cancer actions increases by over 2,000 per cent.[50] In other words, anti-cancer foods work best when combined with other anti-cancer foods.

To highlight the clinical significance of this, consider the following. Researchers aiming to determine the synergistic impacts of anti-cancer nutrition exposed rats to a particularly lethal carcinogen, causing 100 per cent of the rats eating a non-anti-cancer diet to develop cancer. They also gave a cohort of rats exposed to the same carcinogen an anti-cancer diet to follow and in that cohort a significant reduction in cancer was observed. But here comes the crux: as the number of different anti-cancer nutrients they were fed increased, the rates of cancer decreased. In the rats eating only one type of anti-cancer nutrient, a 50 per cent reduction in cancer was observed. In those receiving two anti-cancer nutrients, there was a 66 per cent reduction in cancer. Of the rats that ate all four of the anti-cancer nutrients used in the study, only 10 per cent went on to develop cancer. Thus, in comparison to the 100 per cent of rats that developed cancer upon exposure to the carcinogen without nutritional intervention, a 90 per cent reduction in this risk was induced by a synergistic anti-cancer diet.[51]

While in this example the research was conducted with rats and not humans, it still strongly alludes to the exponentially profound impacts of not just anti-cancer nutrition but synergistic and varied anti-cancer nutrition. This is why adopting the six tastes of Ayurveda is so powerful and so effective: it allows us to harness the power of nutritional synergy in an unparalleled way. And it is also incredibly easy to adopt. Consider the following meal examples, which come from the online Recipes and Meal Plan that accompany this book and can be found at www.mind-body-medical.co.uk/becomingexceptional. These show how effortless it is to use this model to inform a day's worth of tasty and nutritionally dense anti-cancer meals.

**BREAKFAST: ANTI-CANCER OATS**

Wholegrain oats (sweet)
Almond milk (sweet)
Crushed Brazil nuts and almonds (sweet)
Fresh or frozen berries (sour)
A drizzle of lemon (sour)
Finely grated courgette (bitter)
Finely grated fresh ginger (pungent)
½ teaspoon of turmeric powder and black pepper (astringent and pungent)
Hemp seeds (sweet)
Ghee (sweet)
Small pinch of sea salt (salt)
Served with a cup of coffee (bitter), green tea or black tea (astringent)

### LUNCH: HUMMUS, TOASTED WHOLEMEAL PITTA AND STIR-FRIED KALE

- Chickpeas (astringent)
- Extra-virgin olive oil (sweet)
- Turmeric powder (bitter)
- Chilli (pungent)
- Whole tahini paste (sweet)
- Garlic (pungent)
- Lemon juice (sour)
- Rock salt (salt)
- Black pepper (pungent)
- Side serving of stir-fried kale and garlic with pine nuts (bitter and sweet)
- Wholemeal pitta bread (sweet)

### DINNER: SRI LANKAN CHICKPEA SAG CURRY

- Onions (pungent)
- Garlic (pungent)
- Ginger (pungent)
- Chilli (pungent)
- Tomatoes (sour)
- Turmeric (bitter)
- Cayenne pepper (pungent)
- Cinnamon (sweet)
- Rock salt (salt)
- Spinach or chard (bitter)
- Chickpeas (astringent)
- Lime juice (sour)
- Wholegrain rice (sweet)

See how simple this can be? If you add up the collective volume of anti-cancer foods consumed from this day's meal plan, and the way in which they comprehensively address all the primary hallmarks of cancer suppression multiple times over in a synergistic way, we can quickly see why this model of eating is as powerful as it is sustainable.

To get you started in using the six tastes of Ayurveda, you can find a comprehensive meal plan and recipes that contain massive volumes of anti-cancer foods in the aforementioned online Recipes and Meal Plan section. I would recommend using this meal plan not just because the meals taste great but also because it will allow you to build confidence and learn how to modify all your meals to incorporate the six tastes in a practical, long-term and sustainable way.

---

To conclude this chapter, I would like to digress to one final point about the adoption of a robust anti-cancer diet: our subjective interpretation of it. In chapter 3, we explored the importance of our beliefs and the ways in which they can impact upon and alter the physiological workings of the body. Similarly, it is my view that the healing impacts of the food we eat become more pronounced when we become increasingly conscious and aware of these benefits. When you are taking the time to change the way you shop for food and prepare your meals to support healing, and when you sit down with that meal in front of you, why not conclude the process by shutting your eyes and silently acknowledging the healing potential of what you are about to eat? Reaffirm your belief in the ability of food – this plateful of lovingly prepared and unimaginably powerful food in front of you – to nourish your body in truly profound ways as you journey down the road to becoming exceptional. Consciously acknowledge the power and the evidence of nutritional medicine to directly and quantifiably suppress the primary hallmarks of cancer promotion. Before you go to bed tonight, quietly look at yourself in the mirror and recognise that this has been a day well lived. That you have eaten in a way that has saturated your body with an abundance of anti-cancer goodness. That you are empowered. That you are hopeful. And ultimately that you are in control.

##  Chapter Affirmations for My Journey to Becoming Exceptional

1. I acknowledge and recognise the profound healing potential to be found in vibrant and life-giving whole foods.
2. I commit to nourishing my body every day using the full spectrum of foods from all of the six tastes to ensure I am unleashing the full potential of anti-cancer nutritional medicine.
3. As I nourish my body in this way, and acknowledge the accumulative gains it affords me, I will begin to recognise the subtle and progressive changes in my health and energy as I move to a new and vibrant level of health.
4. **Summary Affirmation:** Each and every day I nourish my body with wholefood goodness as a vital part of my journey to becoming exceptional.

## CHAPTER SIX

# Agni and Ojas

### The Elixir of Health and Immunity

*To eat is to be human, but to digest is to be divine.*
AYURVEDIC PROVERB

In the previous chapter we explored in great detail why the optimisation of our diet is of such fundamental importance in the context of cancer survivorship. In this chapter, I would like to progress that exploration in a way that will allow us to further benefit from the anti-cancer dietary modifications we are making. To do that, we need to be aware that *what* we eat constitutes only 50 per cent of the overall nutritional equation. To better understand why this is the case, we can turn to a famous Ayurvedic maxim that is central to unlocking the full and complete benefits of nutritional medicine:

We are not **what** we eat; rather we are what we **digest**.

In other words, to benefit from all of the anti-cancer nutrients found within our food, simply ensuring that we are eating the correct types of food is not enough. This is because nutrients only become health-giving when they are physically extracted from the food that contains them and are effectively delivered into our cells. Until this happens, nutrients are simply molecules with the potential to support healing. To fully and effectively harness this potential, we have to ensure that these nutrients actually reach our cells. This requires an optimally functioning digestive system that is able to effectively extract nutrients from our food and deliver these nutrients into our bloodstream for transportation throughout our body before supporting their final entry across the cell wall and into the cell itself. It is only at this point that the dormant potential of any given anti-cancer nutrient can be fully realised.

A robust anti-cancer diet doesn't begin and end with eating the right foods. It begins with eating the right food and ends with its proper and complete digestion. Viewed through this lens, we can see that our food choices and our digestive capacity are simply different sides of the same anti-cancer dietary coin. And both sides of this coin need to be consciously and proactively attended to in equal measures. In the previous chapter we attended to the *what* to eat. The aim of this chapter is to is to explore how we optimise the *digestion* of what we eat.

Fortunately, Ayurveda has a whole clinical discipline devoted to the topic called *agni deepana*. From the Sanskrit, *agni* translates as 'fire' or 'that which consumes' and relates to the entire workings of the gastrointestinal and metabolic systems of the body, and *deepana* means 'that which kindles'. Thus, the therapeutic modalities of agni deepana involve the kindling of our digestive fire in a way that ensures we realise the full nutritional potential of the food we are eating. The practices of agni deepana are also intimately linked to the promotion of robust immune defence.

In Ayurvedic terminology, the working of the human immune system, in its broadest capacity, is called *ojas*. Ojas is one of the most beautiful and important concepts within the entire framework of Ayurveda and one that is of utmost importance in the context of cancer survivorship. And while ojas includes under its banner everything that Western medicine labels as immunity – our individual immune cells, immune cell production, immune system communication and so on – it is also so much more than that. Ojas is what is responsible for providing us with transformative levels of vitality, energy, strength and vigour, in both body and mind.

Think back to a time in your life when you were absolutely at the highest level of health you have ever experienced. What attributes did you enjoy during that time? Usually it is a sense of vitality and energy, youthfulness, excitement, optimism, strength, healthy-looking skin, hair and eyes, the absence of aches, pains or other symptoms and an over-riding sense of wellbeing. That subjective and objective outpouring of health you just recalled is ojas. When living with cancer and striving to regain optimal health, the conscious cultivation of ojas is a key target. In that capacity, the concept of agni takes centre stage. The aim of the rest of this chapter is to explore the vital and interdependent topics of agni and ojas and to show how together they very much function as a true elixir of health and immunity.

## Agni: The Foundation of Health

The human gastrointestinal and metabolic systems perform an almost unimaginable array of tasks every second of the day in a hugely complex display of physiological regulation. This regulation spans the function of many different organs and areas of the body: the salivary responses in the mouth; the digestive acids and processes found in the stomach; the almost infinitely complex workings of the liver, gall bladder and pancreas; the activity of the small intestine; and finally, the mysterious workings of the colon. And the colon truly is mysterious; it houses the gut microbiome, whose impacts and implications upon the promotion of health, the regulation of healing, and the prevention and management of disease – including cancer – appear to be all-pervading, as we shall see shortly.

In Ayurveda, all these individual but interdependent parts of the gastrointestinal system, from the mouth down to the rectum, fall under the banner of agni. The primary function of agni is to ensure the complete and proper digestion, absorption and assimilation of the nutrients found in the food we eat and the efficient delivery of these nutrients into the tissues and cells of our body. Remember, this is key: anti-cancer nutrients only become so once they actually enter into the cells of the body.

A specific type of agni, called *pilu agni*, is responsible for regulating this process of cellular nutrient delivery. It achieves this by regulating the semi-permeability of our cell walls to allow all the nutritional molecules found circulating in the blood to pass through the cell wall and into the cell itself. It is at this point, and at this point only, that the primary job of agni is completed. For it has succeeded in its ultimate aim of taking the initial unrefined food matter we have eaten and transforming it into superfine particles that can nourish and heal our body at the cellular level. The holy grail of anti-cancer nutrition is the adoption of a robust anti-cancer diet married with a perfectly calibrated digestive system that allows us to take full advantage of the anti-cancer foods we are eating. This is where the proactive targeting of agni takes a central role.

However, agni is also intimately involved in ensuring the optimal workings of another vitally, perhaps centrally, important component of the human digestive system: our gut microbiome. The gut microbiome refers to the colony of trillions of microbes – bacteria, viruses and fungi – that makes up the microbiota that lives in the gut, primarily the colon. Current evidence speculates that there are over 100 trillion microorganisms within the human microbiota, which contain two hundred times more genes than all the genes found in our cells put together.[1] Thus, from an objective perspective, the human body is more microbial in origin than it is mammalian. And this colossal colony of microbes is rapidly being shown to be arguably the single most important factor in determining our health status, why we get sick, what diseases we develop and our ability to recover from these diseases.[2] For example, microbiota health has now been shown to be implicated in the prevention of a huge array of diseases, ranging from cancers and heart diseases to diabetes, depression and Alzheimer's, to name but a few.[3]

The protective mechanisms that the microbiome employs are many and varied and, in many ways, still not fully understood. But the most important of these mechanisms include the optimal modulation of the immune system, the regulation of inflammatory status, ensuring the proper and complete absorption of nutrients, the control of DNA and cellular repair, hormone regulation, the management of bodily homeostasis and much else besides.[4] However, the clinical study of the human microbiome is very much a Pandora's box; each new discovery creates more questions than it does answers. But taken collectively, the evidence ultimately points to one outcome: a healthy microbiome is a prerequisite for a healthy body. Even more so, when it comes to the management of disease, the cultivation of a healthy microbiome is essential. In the specific context of cancer, this is largely, but not exclusively, down to the impact of the microbiome on immune modulation. Around 70 per cent to 80 per cent of our entire immune system is produced within, and regulated by, the gut microbiome.[5] The microbiome is increasingly being shown to directly regulate the ways our immune cells behave specifically within the tumour microenvironment, and thus their ability to be effective in the identification and destruction of cancerous cells.[6] As such, acting in a way that supports optimal microbial health within the gut microbiome needs to be an essential aspect of a robust cancer survivorship protocol.

The key methods for doing so centre upon four key variables:

1. The inclusion of a very broad range of different plant-based whole foods on a daily basis.
2. The daily intake of prebiotic foods, which provide a vital fuel source for the healthy bacteria in the gut.

3. The daily intake of probiotic foods, to help repopulate the gut with more healthy bacteria.
4. The prevention of toxic build-up within the colon.

By following the dietary framework explored in the previous chapter, you will ensure that points one to three are attended to. However, when it comes to the fourth point – the prevention of toxic build-up within the colon – the role of agni is once again key. This is because agni is responsible for preventing the accumulation of toxic waste in the gut by ensuring the full and complete breakdown of the food we eat. In Ayurveda, this build-up of toxic waste within the gut (and elsewhere in the body) is called *ama*, which literally translates from the Sanskrit as 'undigested'. Ama is formed when our digestive capacity is compromised and we are unable to effectively and efficiently digest the food we eat. As a result, a progressively increasing volume of semi-digested food builds up in the gastrointestinal tract, particularly the colon, where it then goes on to rot, putrefy and ferment, leading to the formation of myriad toxic byproducts. In time, this toxic waste goes on to significantly disrupt the workings of the gut microbiome by impairing the proliferation and growth of the healthy microbes that live there. The pathological implications of this are of immense significance in terms of impairing immune status, elevating inflammation and reducing nutrient absorption.

In Ayurveda, this build-up of toxic ama is believed to be the root cause of well over 90 per cent of diseases. The actual word for disease in Sanskrit is *amaya*, which means 'to be born from ama'. But what is so interesting is that in the Ayurvedic concept of ama we find an exact and equal equivalent to the Western state of dysbiosis. Defined as an imbalance in our gut's microorganisms, dysbiosis is characterised by a build-up of pathogenic and disease-forming 'bad' bacteria in the gut microbiome and a corresponding reduction in 'good' bacteria. While there are many variables that can cause dysbiosis, such as certain medications, gastric infections, antibiotics and stress, arguably the most common cause is poor digestive capacity. Or in Ayurvedic parlance, dysfunctional agni. Evidence has shown that factors such as sluggish digestion, reduced digestive enzymes, poor bile production, sluggish bile flow, impaired nutrient breakdown and low stomach acid are all strongly implicated in the development of dysbiosis.[7] And there is now a growing and compelling foundation of clinical evidence to highlight just how dangerous dysbiosis is in relation to the activation of pro-cancer mechanisms in the body. For example, dysbiosis in the gut has been shown to suppress immune activity, reduce circulating immune counts, reduce immune activity specifically within the tumour microenvironment, increase pro-cancer inflammatory markers, reduce DNA repair mechanisms, speed up cancer proliferation rates and aid cancer's ability to evade growth suppressors.[8]

At the time of writing, the clinical focus around the significance and relevance of the gut microbiome upon cancer biology is exploding. As more research is undertaken, we see increasing synergy between the Ayurvedic concept of agni and the Western understanding of the gut microbiome. What this synergy shows is that to exist in a healthy body, a healthy gut and digestive system is not a luxury but a prerequisite. It also shows that to optimise our survivorship potential, acting proactively to cultivate robust digestive and gut health is essential. And to do that, we can call upon the beautifully holistic and individualised therapeutic applications of agni deepana.

## Understanding and Balancing Your Agni

We can now see why it is so crucial that we, as individuals, are empowered with the knowledge needed to cultivate robust and healthy agni. Doing so requires us to firstly understand how to accurately assess the unique and individualised workings of our own agni and, having done so, how to treat and balance it should it display symptoms of dysfunction. However, agni is not dualistic and doesn't function from a place of either balance or imbalance, strength or weakness. Like most things in Ayurveda, it is important to personalise the process and ascertain how your agni is working in relation to you as a unique individual. To do this, we need to briefly revisit the three doshas that we explored in chapter 2 (see Ayurveda: The Science of Optimal Living on page 15).

You will remember that Ayurveda recognises three specific individual mind-body constitutions, called doshas. These are referred to as vata, pitta and kapha. If you have completed the Vikruti Assessment Questionnaire in appendix 1 (where you can also find a weblink to a detailed exploration of the doshas for the interested reader) then you should have a good general understanding of your own current doshic make-up. In the same way that the doshas inform and control every single facet of what makes you 'you' – the colour of your eyes, your personality, your likes and dislikes, your physiological make-up, and all the other myriad physical and psychological variables that constitute you – the doshas also impact upon the state of our agni. So, when our doshas become imbalanced and we experience the build-up of vikruti – the dust on the hard surface of prakruti that we explored on page 16 in Ayurveda: The Science of Optimal Living, chapter 2– this build-up will go on to directly and negatively impact upon the entire workings of our digestive and metabolic systems – our agni. Ayurveda recognises three primary states of dysfunctional agni, which correlate to the three individual doshas. Thus, there is a dysfunctional state of agni that has been negatively affected by vata, a dysfunctional state of agni that has been negatively affected by pitta and a dysfunctional state of agni that has been negatively affected by kapha. Understanding where you, as a unique individual, fall within this framework of agni diagnostics is of fundamental importance in the context of this chapter specifically, this book collectively and the larger focus of exceptional cancer survivorship generically. The following sections provide an in-depth exploration of these three states of agni dysfunction, including how they present, how to diagnose them and, most importantly, how to treat and rebalance them.

### Vata-Imbalanced Agni: The Element of Air

From the Sanskrit, vata translates as 'wind' and this best describes the energising, animating and erratic properties of vata. And because vata is primarily made up of the element of air and wind, we see a particular dominance of these qualities in an agni that has been compromised by vata. The Sanskrit term for a vata-imbalanced agni is *vishama*, which translates as 'irregular digestive fire', and this is exactly how people with this type of digestive function present. If your digestive and metabolic systems have become negatively affected by a build-up of vata, it is likely that you would be experiencing a selection of the following diagnostic characteristics:

| **Primary Digestive Symptoms** | Bloating |
|---|---|
| | Cramping |
| | Wind |
| | Gurgling tummy |
| | Lots of tummy noise |
| | Nervous tummy |

| | |
|---|---|
| **Appetite Presentation** | Very variable<br>Sometimes gets hungry but can sometimes go all day without feeling hungry<br>Usually happy to miss meals |
| **Typical Bowel Function** | Can be prone to constipation<br>Often dryer, harder stools<br>Often rabbit pellet-like stools<br>Bowel movements at varying times of the day |
| **Common Concurrent Physical Symptoms** | Dry skin<br>Dry hair<br>Arthritis<br>Joint pain<br>Osteoporosis<br>Poor circulation<br>Sensitivity to the cold<br>Nerve pain<br>Insomnia/restless sleep |
| **Common Concurrent Emotional Symptoms** | Anxiety<br>Stress<br>Restlessness<br>Insecurity<br>Indecisiveness<br>Fear<br>Excessive multitasking<br>An inability to finish projects and jobs |

Clinical evidence suggests that this is arguably the most common type of digestive imbalance in the West, with most people experiencing many of the cardinal symptoms of a vata-imbalanced agni on a regular basis. However, it is important to emphasise that this type of digestive dysfunction responds very well to treatment and significant improvements can be experienced very quickly after treatment begins.

**Task:** Please spend some time contemplatively considering these symptoms. Don't rush through them but rather use them as a catalyst for cultivating a deeper and more insightful understanding of your digestive system. Think about how your digestive system typically presents. Then think about how it presents after eating foods that perhaps don't agree with you, if you eat too much, too little or at different times of the day, or if you are feeling stressed, anxious and overwhelmed. If you recognise a predominance of these symptoms, then it is very likely that you are experiencing a vata-imbalanced agni. If this is the case, the following section will empower you with a selection of time-tested and proven practices for remedying this situation. And with that comes an increased ability to extract more nutrients from the food you eat, higher levels of gut-based immune function, a healthier microbiome, reduced gut-based toxicity and reduced inflammation throughout the body.

You do not need to use all of the approaches listed at the same time. Rather, I recommend a stepwise approach that starts initially with the adoption of the herbal *churna*, tea blends and dietary modifications (steps 1 to 3). Try using these approaches for three to four weeks to determine how effective they are at resolving the digestive imbalances you are experiencing. If you notice a significant improvement, then simply continue to use these on an ongoing basis. However, if you don't experience enough of an improvement, move on to using the more targeted and powerful approaches (steps 4 to 5) for several weeks; doing so is usually enough to help resolve any stubborn digestive symptoms.

## Treating Vata-Imbalanced Agni

### 1. VATA AGNI-BALANCING HERBAL INFUSION

This vata-balancing herbal tea tastes amazing and can really help to relieve common vata-based digestive symptoms, such as gas, bloating, wind and general digestive discomfort or pain. Use a mortar and pestle for herbs that need to be crushed; they should retain some texture rather than being ground to a powder.

**Ingredients**

2 cardamom pods, gently crushed
½ teaspoon fennel seeds, gently crushed
1 small cinnamon stick
½ teaspoon finely grated fresh ginger
squeeze of lemon juice

**Method:** To make the tea, simply add all the ingredients into a teapot or jug, pour on a cupful of boiling water and leave to steep for ten minutes.

Strain the infusion through a tea strainer or fine-mesh sieve into a cup when it's ready. You should drink one cup an hour before each meal and again at any time that suits you in the evening.

### 2. VATA AGNI-BALANCING CHURNA

A churna is an Ayurvedic pre-blended herbal mix that is added to food and cooking as a way of not just increasing flavour but also to support optimal digestion. The recipe below is designed to specifically balance a digestion that is being negatively affected by vata. Having used this churna with hundreds of patients over the years, I have seen it transform gut health and I can't recommend it enough. All the culinary herbs it contains are proven in their capacity to support optimal digestive function.

**Ingredients**

8 teaspoons cumin seeds
8 teaspoons fennel seeds
2 teaspoons coriander seeds
2 teaspoons turmeric powder
1 teaspoon ginger powder
¼ teaspoon cinnamon powder

**Method:** Put all the ingredients into a coffee grinder, NutriBullet or other electric grinder and grind to a fine powder. If you don't have access to an electric grinder, you can crush the herbs into a fine powder using a mortar and pestle. Decant the ground mixture into a clean, dry jar with an airtight lid and store it in a cool place away from direct sunlight.

**How to Use:** Add the churna to your meal as part of the cooking process to allow the digestion-balancing compounds in the herbs to enter the food. This helps to support the more effective breakdown and digestion of the food after eating it. How much churna you need to use depends on both your personal taste and the type of dish you are making. For example, for a robust dish such as curry that you are cooking for six people, half a teaspoon per person is fine; however, for a lighter dish this could be too overpowering, and you may want to reduce the amount of churna used. As you cook more with churnas, you will learn what quantities work best for you; it is fine to start by using a little less and build up to more as you discover how different flavours work with your churna. For foods cooked in water or a sauce (for example vegetables, rice, pasta, grains, soups and curries), simply mix the churna into the water or sauce at the start of the cooking process. If you are cooking your food in fat (as with fried, roasted, marinated or baked dishes), melt the cooking fat, such as ghee or coconut oil, in your pan or roasting tin, then stir in your churna before adding the rest of your ingredients.

### 3. DIETARY MODIFICATIONS

In the previous chapter we explored the six tastes of Ayurveda. Of these there are three tastes that are specifically indicated for balancing vata and three that when eaten in excess can further aggravate it. The three tastes that balance vata are the anabolic (sweet), salty and sour tastes, while the bitter, pungent and astringent tastes can exacerbate vata. If you are experiencing a vata-imbalanced agni, it is still absolutely vital that you include all six tastes in your daily diet. However, you should also put more emphasis on the anabolic tastes as these are the most effective foods for balancing vata. Likewise, ensure the sour and salty tastes are present in every meal. In contrast, try to slightly reduce the volume of bitter, pungent and astringent foods in your meals until the digestive symptoms you are experiencing begin to ease. Also try to ensure that the bitter, astringent and pungent foods that you do eat are warm and cooked rather than eaten cold or raw.

### 4. VATA AGNI-BALANCING CULINARY HERBS

Aside from using the more concentrated Vata Agni-Balancing Churna, seasoning and flavouring your meals with an abundance of herbs and spices can make a tremendous difference to nutrient assimilation, digestion and gut health. Furthermore, the concentrations of active anti-cancer compounds found in these types of culinary herbs are incredibly dense, and they make a fantastic and easy way of further topping up your daily intake of anti-cancer dietary compounds. The list below provides an overview of which herbs have a particular affinity for balancing and remedying vata-based digestive symptoms:

| | | |
|---|---|---|
| Ginger | Cloves | Fenugreek |
| Cumin | Nutmeg | Turmeric |
| Black pepper | Paprika | Fennel |
| Sea or rock salt | Bay leaves | Mustard seeds |

**5. VATA AGNI-TARGETING HERBAL MEDICINES**

If the preceding approaches fail to remedy your vata-based digestive symptoms within three to four weeks of use, the following herbs provide a much more targeted, powerful and specific impact on regulating vata-based digestion.

**i. Hing:** This incredibly powerful herb, usually called asafoetida in the West, represents arguably the single most effective vata-balancing digestive herb of them all. Often referred to as 'devil's dung' due to its strong aroma, it is a staple in most traditional Ayurvedic cooking. This is because of the profound impact it can have upon the management of vata-induced digestive symptoms, such as bloating, cramping, gastric spasms, gas, flatulence, colic and weak digestion. In this capacity, it is truly unrivalled. However, it is a very strong herb and only needs to be used in small amounts – ideally 100 milligrams per day added into cooking. To use, simply add a small pinch into curries, casseroles, stews or dhals – in fact, almost any recipe – to tap into all its many potent benefits. But a word of caution: because of its heating and gut-stimulating properties, it is not to be used in those experiencing inflammatory gut disorders such as gastritis, acidity, reflux, heartburn, peptic ulcers, colitis or Crohn's disease.

**ii. Tulsi:** Another key Ayurvedic tonic herb, tulsi is an incredibly effective and warming digestive stimulant that helps to increase appetite, stimulate digestion, support the breakdown and assimilation of nutrients, and generally balance vata-imbalanced agni. Also known as holy basil, tulsi possesses revered anti-spasmodic properties, which excel in their ability to alleviate the primary vata-based digestive symptoms, such as cramping, gastric spasms, bloating, distension and wind. In the context of supporting digestion, it is best to take tulsi as a herbal tea. One tulsi teabag can be added to the Vata Agni-Balancing Herbal Infusion recipe on page 101, or simply aim to drink one to two cups of tulsi tea per day. Tulsi tea can be sourced from the Herbal Medicines suppliers listed in appendix 3 (see page 227).

## Pitta-Imbalanced Agni: The Element of Fire

Having discussed vata agni, we will now look to the assessment and treatment of pitta, the second dosha. *Pitta* translates from the Sanskrit as 'that which transforms', which perfectly encapsulates the metabolising, transforming, converting, digesting and chemically modifying properties of pitta. In the context of agni regulation, pitta has a central role as it is directly involved in the control and management of our entire digestive system collectively. The very word pitta comes from the root 'tap', which means 'to cook or transform'. When visualising the role of pitta, it is often easiest to think of it as the 'fire' in the body, just as we thought of vata as being the 'air/wind' in the body. The Ayurvedic term for an agni that has been negatively affected by pitta is *tikshna*, which translates as 'a sharp, insatiable and penetrating fire', which is precisely how people with this digestive function present. If your digestive and metabolic systems are being negatively affected by a build-up of pitta, you will probably be experiencing a range of the following diagnostic features:

| | |
|---|---|
| **Primary Digestive Symptoms** | Acidity<br>Heartburn<br>Reflux<br>Peptic ulcers<br>Hypoglycaemia<br>Very fast metabolism |
| **Appetite Presentation** | Strong appetite<br>Often feels hungry<br>Hates to miss meals or eat later than planned<br>Can typically eat large portions |
| **Typical Bowel Function** | Can be prone to loose stools<br>Multiple bowel movements each day<br>Acute aggravations can cause diarrhea<br>Yellowy, often burning stools |
| **Common Concurrent Physical Symptoms** | Inflammatory bowel diseases such as gastritis, Crohn's disease, colitis and diverticulitis<br>Mouth ulcers<br>Eczema, hives and skin rashes<br>Spots and acne<br>Feeling hot, high body temperature<br>Excess sweating or sweats easily<br>Hair loss/thinning hair<br>Hormone problems |

| | |
|---|---|
| **Common Concurrent Emotional Symptoms** | Anger |
| | Irritability |
| | Short-temperedness |
| | Impatience |
| | Judgemental |
| | Critical of others |
| | Perfectionist |
| | Hostility |
| | Obsessiveness |
| | Domineering |
| | Intolerant |

**Task:** As with the assessment of vata agni, please take time to contemplatively consider these symptoms. If you recognise a predominance of these symptoms relevant to those associated with a vata- or kapha-compromised agni, then it is very likely that you are experiencing a pitta-imbalanced agni. If this is true for you, the proven and well-established practices in the following sections will enable you to remedy this condition. As with addressing vata-imbalanced agni, begin with steps 1 to 3, but if you find you aren't improving enough, move on to steps 4 and 5 as well.

## Treating Pitta-Imbalanced Agni

### 1. PITTA AGNI-BALANCING HERBAL INFUSION

This pitta-specific herbal tea is incredibly cooling to both body and mind. And as well as tasting amazing, it can really help to relieve common pitta-based digestive symptoms, particularly heartburn, acidity and reflux. It is also very effective for inflammatory gut ailments, such as peptic ulcers, gastritis and colitis. To crush the herbs, use a mortar and pestle to break them up while avoiding grinding them to a powder.

### Ingredients

½ teaspoon fennel seeds, gently crushed

1 to 2 cardamom pods, gently crushed

1 teaspoon fresh or dried mint *or* 1 mint teabag

**Method:** Put all the ingredients into a jug or teapot. Add a cupful of boiling water and leave the mixture to steep for ten minutes. Once ready, strain the tea into a mug; drink one cup an hour before each meal and one more in the evening.

## 2. PITTA AGNI-BALANCING CHURNA

As previously discussed, a churna is an Ayurvedic pre-blended herbal mix that you add to food and cooking to increase flavour and support optimal digestion. The following recipe will specifically balance a negatively affected digestion that is being caused by pitta dosha.

**Ingredients**

10 teaspoons fennel seeds
2 teaspoons coriander seeds
2 teaspoons turmeric powder

**Method:** Grind all the herbs to a fine powder using a coffee grinder or electric grinder such as a NutriBullet. If you don't have an electric grinder, this can be done in a mortar and pestle. Then decant the powder into a clean, dry jar with an airtight lid. Store the churna away from sunlight in a dry, cool place.

**How to Use:** To allow the digestion-balancing compounds in the herbs to combine with your food, you should add the churna to your ingredients as part of the cooking process. This enables you to more effectively break down and digest your food. As discussed in the Vata Agni-Balancing Churna, how much churna you use will depend on the dish you are cooking and your own personal tastes, though this is usually around half to one teaspoon per person. As you cook more with churna, you will get to know how much to use in the foods you make. For foods such as vegetables, rice, pasta, grains, soups and curries that are cooked in water or sauce, simply mix the churna into the water or sauce at the beginning of the cooking process. For fried, roasted, marinated or baked dishes that are cooked in fat, first melt the cooking fat in your pan or roasting tin, then stir in your churna. Add the rest of the ingredients and cook as required.

## 3. DIETARY MODIFICATIONS

As we explored during our discussion of how to balance vata agni, three of the six tastes of Ayurveda are specifically recommended for balancing pitta and three can, in excess, further aggravate pitta. The three tastes that balance pitta are the anabolic (sweet), bitter and astringent tastes, while excess pungent, salty and sour tastes can further inflame it. If you are experiencing a pitta-imbalanced agni, it is still essential for you to include all six tastes in your daily diet. However, it is also important to try to ensure that your meals contain a higher volume of foods from the anabolic, bitter and astringent tastes. In contrast, try to reduce the volume of pungent, sour and salty foods in each meal until the digestive symptoms you are experiencing ease.

### 4. PITTA AGNI-BALANCING CULINARY HERBS

As well as using the more concentrated Pitta Agni-Balancing Churna, adding a selection of pitta-balancing culinary herbs into your cooking and meal preparation can really help to support a digestive system that has been aggravated by pitta. The herbs listed here are especially efficacious for this.

| Mint | Coriander; leaves | Cardamom |
|---|---|---|
| Rosemary | and seeds | Fennel |
| Basil | Parsley | |
| Saffron | Turmeric | |

### 5. PITTA AGNI-TARGETING HERBAL MEDICINES: AMLA

If within three to four weeks of use none of the previous approaches remedy your symptoms, the famous and much revered Ayurvedic tonic amla – *amalaki* in Sanskrit – excels in its ability to bring balance to pitta-based digestive symptoms. Amla helps to optimise appetite, digestion and the assimilation of nutrients to ensure we extract maximal benefit from the food we eat. Furthermore, amla is one of the most incredibly cooling and anti-inflammatory herbs in the world, indicating its use in the management of the common pitta-based inflammatory digestive problems, such as acidity, acid reflux, heartburn, gastritis, colitis, Crohn's disease, peptic ulcers, inflammatory bowel syndrome (IBS) and general inflammatory bowel disease. To benefit from amla's digestion-optimising and anti-inflammatory abilities, it is recommended to take it in juice form, ideally drinking 30 to 40 millilitres twice daily. Please see the herbal suppliers listed under Herbal Medicines in appendix 3 (page 227) for where to source certified amla juice.

## Kapha-Imbalanced Agni: The Element of Earth

We now turn our attention to the third and final dosha, kapha. Conceptually speaking, *kapha* translates as 'that which protects, nourishes and holds things together', which excellently describes the strengthening, stabilising, lubricating, cushioning, protecting and supporting roles that kapha plays in the body. Kapha makes up the bulk of the human body in terms of the physical structures of our cells, tissues, bones, muscles, bodily fluids and organs. It is also responsible for nourishing these tissues with the correct nutrients to ensure optimal health. Crucially, kapha is also heavily involved in the function of the immune and lymphatic systems, which, as we have seen, play a vital role in our body's inherent anti-cancer defences. The Ayurvedic term for an agni that has been negatively affected by kapha is *manda*, which translates as 'a slow-burning and sluggish fire'. And that is precisely how this type of digestive function manifests. If a build-up of kapha is the reason why your digestive and metabolic systems have become negatively affected, you will likely be experiencing a number of the following symptoms:

| | |
|---|---|
| **Primary Digestive Symptoms** | Slow metabolism |
| | Fatigue and tiredness after eating |
| | Slow to digest food |
| | Sense of food 'sitting' in the stomach and taking a long time to be cleared |
| | Tendency to over-eat |
| | Gains weight very easily |
| | Finds it hard to lose weight |
| **Appetite Presentation** | Very uncommon to experience physical sensations of hunger |
| | Never hungry in the morning |
| | Despite this, it is common to over-eat |
| **Typical Bowel Function** | Bowel movement most days |
| | Stools often quite sticky |
| | Usually lots of stool |
| | Can be oily and/or with mucus |

| | |
|---|---|
| **Common Concurrent Physical Symptoms** | Being over-weight/obesity<br>Type 2 diabetes<br>High cholesterol<br>Water retention<br>Mucus congestion<br>Respiratory problems<br>Allergies<br>Gall stones<br>Heavy menstrual cycles |
| **Common Concurrent Emotional Symptoms** | Emotional/comfort eating<br>Cognitive and emotional lethargy<br>Despondency<br>Sluggishness<br>Drowsiness<br>Depression and low mood<br>Feeling flat<br>Mental fogginess<br>Lacking motivation<br>Withdrawal |

**Task:** As suggested for vata and pitta agni, spend some time contemplatively considering these types of kapha-based agni presentations. If you recognise a predominance of these symptoms then it is very likely that you are experiencing a kapha-imbalanced agni. In this case, what follows are some tried and tested approaches that have been shown to address this situation. Just as with treating the other agni imbalances, start with steps 1 to 3, and move on to steps 4 and 5 if you feel like you need more help in improving.

## Balancing Kapha-Imbalanced Agni
### 1. KAPHA AGNI-BALANCING HERBAL INFUSION
This herbal tea is an incredibly well-known and effective kapha-stimulating blend, which can really help to relieve common kapha-based digestive symptoms, particularly those that present with low appetite, sluggish digestion and weight gain. It is also effective for remedying other non-gut-based kapha ailments, such as respiratory congestion, fatigue and a general lack of vitality

and 'get-up-and-go'. It is best to use a mortar and pestle to crush the herbs for this recipe, so that they don't get ground into a powder.

**Ingredients**

1 teaspoon cumin seeds, gently crushed
1 teaspoon coriander seeds, gently crushed
1 teaspoon fennel seeds, gently crushed
2 teaspoons finely grated fresh ginger
3 whole cloves, gently crushed
1 cinnamon stick

**Method:** Pour 1 litre of water into a saucepan, add all the herbs and then bring the liquid to a boil. Remove the pan from the heat and allow the infusion to steep for ten minutes. Strain the liquid into a jug, then pour it into a thermos. Take frequent sips throughout the day – ideally, at least a couple of sips every thirty minutes.

## 2. KAPHA AGNI-BALANCING CHURNA

As with the vata and pitta agni-balancing churnas, this Ayurvedic herbal mix will support optimal digestion and also make your food taste even more flavourful. This recipe will help to balance a digestion that is being negatively affected by kapha.

**Ingredients**

6 teaspoons cumin seeds
6 teaspoons coriander seeds
3 teaspoons turmeric powder
2 teaspoons fenugreek seeds
¼ teaspoon ground ginger
¼ teaspoon black peppercorns

**Method:** Add all the herbs to an electric grinder, such as a NutriBullet, or a coffee grinder and grind until you have a fine powder. You can also do this in a mortar and pestle. Store the powder in a clean, dry jar with an airtight lid in a cool place and away from direct sunlight.

**How to Use:** Use about half to one teaspoon of the churna per person, depending on what kind of dish you are making. As discussed previously, you will learn what suits your tastes and how much churna to add to different foods the more you cook with churnas; for lighter dishes, you may want to use a little less and for more full-flavoured dishes you may add more. If you are cooking your food in water or a sauce, mix the churna into this before adding the rest of the ingredients. For food cooked in fat, melt the fat in your pan or roasting tin, then add the churna and mix it with the fat before adding the rest of your ingredients. Cook your dish as normal. Adding the churna as part of the cooking process means the digestion-balancing properties from these herbs are at their most effective as the compounds are able to combine with your food.

### 3. DIETARY MODIFICATIONS

Of the six tastes of Ayurveda, there are three that are specifically indicated for balancing kapha and three that can exacerbate it if eaten in excess. The three tastes that balance kapha are the pungent, bitter and astringent tastes, while the anabolic (sweet), salty and sour tastes can further aggravate it. If you are experiencing a kapha-imbalanced agni, it is still absolutely vital that you include all of these six tastes in your daily diet. However, also ensure that your meals contain a higher volume of foods from the pungent, bitter and astringent tastes. Conversely, attempt to reduce how much anabolic (sweet), sour and salty foods are in each meal until your digestive symptoms start to improve.

### 4. KAPHA AGNI-BALANCING CULINARY HERBS

Increasing the volume and variety of kapha-balancing culinary herbs that you include in your cooking and meal preparation can really help to support a digestive system that has been aggravated by kapha. The following herbs are particularly effective in this respect:

| Ginger | Turmeric | Nutmeg |
| --- | --- | --- |
| Fennel | Cinnamon | Paprika |
| Black pepper | Cloves | Basil |
| Coriander | Mustard seeds | Chilli |

### 5. KAPHA AGNI-TARGETING HERBAL MEDICINES: TRIKATU

If your kapha-based digestive symptoms still persist after three to four weeks of following the first four approaches, the Ayurvedic herbal formulation trikatu can work wonders. Trikatu is made from equal parts of three dried herbs: black pepper, long pepper and ginger. (Long pepper, often called 'pippali', is a beautifully aromatic type of pepper that grows in the tropical regions of India.) These powerful and pungent herbs excel in their ability to stimulate the slow, heavy and sluggish qualities of kapha-dominant agni. Furthermore, all three of the herbs that make up trikatu have proven anti-cancer benefits, making this a fantastic tonic herb. To harness these benefits, it is recommended to take around 2,000 milligrams per day, ideally taken as 1,000 milligrams in the morning and another 1,000 milligrams in the evening. Please refer to Herbal Medicines on page 227 in appendix 3 for a list of recommended suppliers.

## Agni, Ojas and the Elixir of Health and Immunity

Now that we have discussed how you can assess your unique digestive profile and how to balance this using the practices of agni deepana, there is one absolutely vital concept left for us to explore: ojas. As we have briefly discussed, ojas relates to the Ayurvedic understanding of immunity, but in a much broader and more inclusive way, and it underpins the very foundations of health.

In the *Charaka Samhita*, the most sacred clinical treatise on Ayurveda, it is stated that when the quantity of ojas diminishes too much, life itself is threatened. In contrast, when ojas is abundant, it is responsible for the cultivation of optimal levels of immunity, disease resistance, strength, vigour and robustness in the physical body and an all-pervading sense of positivity, contentment, optimism and empowerment in the emotional and psychological body. It should come as no surprise, then, that in the framework of healing the proactive cultivation of ojas is of fundamental importance. This is true when targeting healing in every sense of the word. But in the specific context of cancer, which by definition is characterised as a weakening of the body and immune system, the building of ojas takes on an even greater level of significance. Because of this, cultivating robust levels of ojas is viewed as a crucial clinical target in the Ayurvedic understanding of cancer survivorship.

And it is agni that acts as the primary lynchpin for doing so. This is because in Ayurvedic physiology, ojas is viewed as the metabolic end product of the complete digestion of the food we eat. So, the food we consume each day goes through a progressively refined state of digestion until, at the very end of this process, the super-refined and digested nutrient load is finally converted in ojas. Thus, to cultivate transformative levels of ojas, we firstly have to prioritise the optimal workings of our digestive and metabolic systems. This is one of the reasons why we should all spend time mindfully assessing the state of our agni and acting to correct any imbalances we find, as explored above.

While the cultivation of high levels of ojas is an integral part of the Ayurvedic understanding of health promotion and disease management, it perhaps takes on an even greater mantle of responsibility when we view it through the lens of Western physiology. For when we do that, we see compelling evidence to suggest that what Ayurveda is talking about when it talks about ojas may, in part, relate directly to the famous hormone melatonin. If this is so, the implications are of profound importance in the arena of cancer survivorship due to the significant and multifactorial role that melatonin plays in the suppression of cancer cell biology. So, before we look at some simple practices for building higher levels of ojas, let us briefly explore this important marriage of ancient and modern in a little more detail.

### Ojas as Melatonin: Why It Matters

Because of the central importance of ojas in the context of health promotion and disease management, there has been extensive debate in both Ayurvedic and Western circles around what ojas actually is. Is it a yet-to-be-identified neurotransmitter? Is it a refined derivative of a specific hormone? Is it a more esoteric and undefinable energy that science has yet to understand? These questions have been asked and debated for decades. But a very clear answer emerges when we try to understand ojas by asking a more practical question: 'What is the closest functional Western equivalent to it?' And that answer is the ubiquitous hormone melatonin. Most of us know of melatonin as the 'sleep' hormone, which it very much is. But this is an incredibly limited view, for in many ways melatonin is a hormonal conductor that controls the orchestra of the human body at myriad levels.

So how, why and in what ways does melatonin relate to ojas? If we look at the Ayurvedic understanding of ojas, it is defined as a superfine biological substance that pervades the workings of the entire body and every cell within it. Similarly, it is responsible for cultivating immunity, health, strength, vigour, contentment and happiness, the ability to prevent disease and the successful management of disease should it occur. If we correlate this definition with the workings of melatonin, we see an almost exact mirror image. Melatonin is a superfine biological substance (as are all hormones) that pervades the entire body and every cell within it, as does ojas. Evidence now shows that *every* cell in the human body has a neuroreceptor for, and is thus directly influenced by, melatonin. Furthermore, melatonin has been shown to exist not just in a cell, but in virtually every part of it, including the cell membrane, cytoplasm, mitochondria and right into the very nucleus of the cell itself, as does ojas.[9] Similarly, if we can compare the roles that melatonin plays within the regulation of our physiology relevant to ojas we see a definitive correlation, as we shall see next.

## Immune Status

At the base level, ojas relates to the capacity and strength of our immune system in Ayurvedic physiology. Similarly, Western clinical evidence shows that melatonin plays an instrumental role in the regulation of the human immune system.[10] Of even more significance is the fact that melatonin has been shown to directly and specifically regulate the activity of key cancer-targeting immune cells directly within the tumour microenvironment.[11] This immune-modulating activity of melatonin has been shown to help suppress cancer cell growth and proliferation in a wide variety of cancers. This indicates the role of melatonin in both the prevention and management of malignant diseases in exactly the same way that is attributed to ojas.

## Physical Energy, Strength and Vigour

As we have seen, ojas is said to increase our levels of physical vitality, energy, strength and vigour. In Western physiological parlance, such qualities are largely attributed to a chemical called adenosine triphosphate (ATP). This is very much the energy currency of the body, whose job it is to store energy and then deliver it into the cells when it is needed. When we lack physical energy, vigour and vitality, it largely (but not exclusively) due to the fact that the body is having difficulty in producing enough ATP. Evidence now shows that melatonin is absolutely vital for the proper and complete synthesis of ATP, and that optimal melatonin levels are a prerequisite for optimum ATP production and thus the cultivation of higher levels of physical energy and vitality.[12] So whether we view this through the lens of East or West, we see the same outcome: to experience the high levels of vitality, energy, strength and vigour we all desire, optimal levels of ojas/melatonin are essential.

### Emotional Health and Vitality

The final primary role played by ojas (there are hundreds of additional roles that go beyond the scope and aims of this book) is to support health and vitality in our emotional body. Living with robust levels of physical health is largely pointless if we lack a corresponding level of joy, happiness and contentment in our emotional body, for these are the psychological traits that make life so magical. Ayurvedically speaking, ojas plays an instrumental role in the cultivation of such traits. So, too, does melatonin. This is because melatonin is intimately involved in the production and regulation of dopamine in the brain.[13] As we know, dopamine is often called our 'happy hormone' due to the central role it plays in our mental and emotional health and preventing states such as depression and anxiety. Indeed, it is now understood that for this reason, melatonin levels are directly linked to our levels of happiness. Thus, in this third and final connection, we see clear synergy between the Ayurvedic view of ojas and the Western view of melatonin.

Either way, when applied to the arena of exceptional cancer survivorship, we can see why the conscious and proactive cultivation of robust levels of ojas is so vitally important; it optimises and regulates cancer-specific immune activation, it improves our levels of physical vitality, vigour and energy, and it helps us experience life through the lens of optimism, positivity and contentment (the importance of which we explored in chapter 3).

## Practical Approaches for Building Robust Ojas

Fortunately, there are many simple and easy-to-implement practices that we can integrate into our life in a way that will support the production of higher levels of ojas. While most activities that we find uplifting, such as beautiful views, moving music and creative pursuits, hobbies and passions, will help build ojas, the following provides an overview of the key ojas-building practices to adopt:

### Balance Agni

As we have seen, ojas is primarily produced as the end product of the complete and proper digestion of the food we eat. As such, attending to our agni in such a way as to keep it balanced and optimal, using the approaches outlined in this chapter, represents the first, foundational and most important approach for cultivating high levels of ojas.

## Ojas-Building Foods

In addition to the cultivation of ojas via the complete digestion of our food, Ayurveda also advocates the judicious use of 'high-ojas' foods in our diet. These are foods that help to naturally and, in many cases, powerfully increase the levels of ojas in the body. Such foods are classically anabolic and strengthening by nature and dovetail perfectly with the anti-cancer foods explored in the previous chapter. Some of the best ojas-boosting foods include dates, nuts, seeds, ghee, extra-virgin olive oil and coconut oil, honey, bananas, figs, sweet fruits, dairy and nut milks, and wholegrains. Interestingly, many of these high-ojas foods are also naturally high in melatonin. As well as including these foods in our diet, we can also utilise them in a more concentrated manner. To facilitate this, please refer to the High Ojas Recipe Bundle, which can be found in the Recipes and Meal Plan section of the online resources that accompany this book: www.mind-body-medical.co.uk/becomingexceptional. There you will find a variety of incredibly tasty, nutritious and ojas-dense snacks and drinks. These are fantastic options to integrate into your daily life, especially if you are looking to increase your overall levels of energy and vitality or if you need to proactively attend to increasing or maintaining your body weight.

## Ojas-Building Lifestyle Practices

Above and beyond attending to our diet and digestion, there are also a variety of lifestyle practices that play an integral role in the building of higher levels of ojas. The most important of these include meditation and contemplative practices (see How to Meditate on page 41 in chapter 3), and the daily self-care practices explored in chapter 8. Ensuring the integration of such practices into your daily life needs to become a key aspect of your overarching cancer survivorship framework.

## Chapter Affirmations for My Journey to Becoming Exceptional

1. I consciously acknowledge the importance of cultivating robust agni as a vital component in my journey back to optimal health.
2. I commit to cultivating mindful daily awareness of my agni and, should I notice a move away from balance, I will acknowledge my ability to rectify this using the transformative practices of agni deepana.

3. I recognise the profound role played by ojas in my quest to become exceptional and commit to the adoption of daily practices that will allow me to enjoy the fruits of robust levels of ojas.
4. I think back to a time in my life when I was experiencing radiant levels of ojas and I sincerely believe in my ability to experience that same level of health, vitality and wellness once again.
5. **Summary Affirmation:** Each and every day I unleash the transformative powers of agni and ojas into my life as I powerfully and purposefully progress along the path of becoming exceptional.

# CHAPTER SEVEN

# Nature's Pharmacy
## Anti-Cancer Herbal Medicines

> *Rejoice, plants bearing abundant flowers, fruits and medicines which triumph over disease like victorious horses, bearing humanity safe beyond the reach of illness and decay.*
>
> Rig Veda

Once upon a time, around 180,000 years ago, a new species of primate emerged on the plains of East Africa. Walking on two legs as opposed to four and covered only very lightly with hair, this new species was distinctly different to the other primates of the time. It possessed a much slighter build and, through an unimaginably complex sequence of evolutionary events, was fortunate to possess a disproportionately large and powerful brain. One day, walking across the pristine savannahs of Tanzania, one particularly curious member of this new species of primate – the species we now call humans – noticed a huge bull elephant gorging on the leaves of a yet unknown and unidentified tree. Our curious forebear watched as the elephant relentlessly ate mouthful after mouthful of the shiny green leaves until the tree was almost bare. Realising how unusual this behaviour was and wondering why the elephant was acting in this way, our forebear decided to follow the elephant. Around an hour later, he noticed something equally unusual: the elephant was rendered virtually immobile as he passed bowel movement after bowel movement. Within two hours of eating the leaves of this obviously important tree, copious volumes of elephant dung littered the ground in a way this early human had never seen before. And then, as the sun began to set, the elephant finally moved on, rejoining his herd to continue grazing as normal. Using the unparalleled deductive powers of his new *Homo sapiens* super-brain, our curious forefather asked a question that would ultimately go on to develop the entire field of clinical medical research: Why? Why had the elephant behaved this way? Why did those specific leaves induce such violent bowel movements? Why not another type of tree? Why had the elephant voluntarily chosen to do this?

These questions, and the curiosity they engendered, ultimately led to the first scientific study ever conducted by our species, for it prompted this early human to go over to the same tree and copy the elephant. He picked the leaves, tore them up into smaller pieces and put them in his mouth and chewed them. He consciously noted the overwhelming bitterness of the leaves and the way it caused saliva to build in his mouth. He then swallowed them. He repeated this until he had eaten a few handfuls of leaves and then observed what happened. He noticed an initial sense of mild nausea in his gut. He noticed the noise and grumbling coming from his tummy. He felt minor cramps in his bowels. And then, as had happened to the elephant, around an hour later this early human experienced an aggressive laxative response. He saw how his stool had taken a more liquid form. He noticed the increased volume of stool he passed and, by the end of the experiment, had learned that this particular tree could be purposefully used by his tribe as a medicine. He learned that should he or someone in his community suffer with the inability to pass stool – what we now call constipation – he could prescribe this unique leaf to help resolve the issue and stored this new information in the powerful brain he benefited from. And thus medicine was practised for the first time. For what this very first healer in the history of our species had discovered on the plains of Tanzania was the senna tree, a herb that is now one of the most widely used medicines in the world for treating constipation.

While we will of course never know exactly how the first humans discovered the use of herbal medicines, medical anthropologists widely acknowledge that it would almost certainly have been in a similar way to that described above. And once it began, it unleashed a torrent of progress as humans desired to learn more about what other plants could be pressed into healing service in this way. What ensued was a systematic process of trial and error as different plants, leaves, fruits, berries, barks and roots were eaten and the subsequent responses observed and memorised.

As the human species flourished and subsequent generations began their slow migration out of the cradle of humanity in East Africa, the foundation of knowledge relating to which plants possessed healing powers and how to harness these was passed down in an unbroken oral tradition. As our species grew into larger and more complex societies, specialised roles emerged, such as those skilled in hunting, tracking and tool building, for example. One such speciality was the emergence of dedicated medicine men and women. Often called shamans, these healers amalgamated all of the medical knowledge passed down to them into a systematic framework of medicine, which they used in their quest to optimise the health of their community and alleviate suffering and disease.

As humanity continued its slow migration into Asia and Europe, the study and application of plant medicine developed accordingly as new plants and herbs, in new ecological environments, were encountered. Thus, an ever-expanding repository of geographically specific knowledge around the application of herbal medicine was developed. And then, somewhere around the period 4000–6000 BCE in the Indus valley of India, this embryonic field of herbal medicine collided with the newly developing science of life that we today call Ayurveda. This collision created the first, oldest and most beautifully holistic treaty on herbal medicine ever recorded, as documented in the *Charaka Samhita*, the definitive clinical text in Ayurveda. This beautiful series of books contains detailed descriptions of myriad different herbal medicines and how best to prepare and use them to preserve health and treat disease. The application of herbal medicine employed by Ayurveda in this way has an unbroken lineage of use that continues right up to the present day and affords us access to a profound level of healing.

As the healers and alchemists of India travelled west into Europe, this knowledge of herbal medicine would, in turn, greatly influence the practitioners of Greek medicine such as Hippocrates and Galen, who are recognised as being the founding fathers of the modern allopathic medicine we enjoy today. This unstoppable progression of herbal medicine continued in different guises over the ensuing centuries until it moved into the evidence-based movement that is the hallmark of medical research in the twentieth and twenty-first centuries.

Over the last several decades, the traditional practices of herbal medicine have been subjected to intense and robust clinical investigation. What this investigation has revealed, and continues to reveal right up to the present day, is that herbal medicines possess an unimaginably powerful and often unique capacity to alter the physiological workings of the body in the direction of healing. This is true of all healing in all contexts. For example, there is peer-reviewed published evidence to show that herbal medicines offer clinical efficacy in managing everything from high blood pressure and diabetes to Alzheimer's disease and arthritis, and virtually everything in between. Fortunately for us, the research emerging specifically within the arena of cancer is no different.

During the last twenty years, there has been an explosion of clinical research into the anti-cancer impacts of a huge array of both Ayurvedic and non-Ayurvedic herbs. What this research shows is that these herbs possess immense potential to support the collective health and wellbeing of those living with cancer. But so often this potential remains unknown and untapped by those who need it the most. The aim of this chapter is to provide a framework for remedying this problem by providing a clear and evidence-based exploration of a selection of the most important anti-cancer herbs available to us: how they work, the evidence to support them and how best to use them, along with a full discussion of the safety implications of doing so. The hope being that by the end of this chapter you will be inspired, empowered and motivated to begin exploring the use of herbal medicines with your clinical care team as an integral aspect of your overall cancer survivorship blueprint.

## Herbs as Medicine

At the very foundational level it is a commonsensical but often overlooked fact that our very existence is dependent upon the vegetable kingdom and the plants, trees and herbs it contains. Without the vegetable kingdom's ability to transform sunlight into the catalyst for the growth of all of the fruits and vegetables we need to stay healthy we would never have developed or survived as a species. At the even more foundational level, we are completely and wholly dependent upon the vegetable kingdom for every single lungful of life-preserving oxygen we breathe. But above and beyond these prerequisites of survival, the vegetable kingdom is also responsible for gifting us the vast majority of the medicines we use to preserve health and treat disease.

From a conventional point of view, around 70 per cent of the pharmaceutical drugs employed by Western medicine are derived from plants.[1] Similarly, across the entire human population, traditional herbal medicine is still the most widely used form of healthcare on the planet, supporting the health of over 80 per cent of the world's population every year.[2] We can very clearly see from these statistics that when it comes to the cultivation of health and the management of disease, the vegetable kingdom is one of our most powerful allies and providers.

Western clinical research has fortunately been very quick to acknowledge this fact and the last several decades have seen an exponential increase in the number of clinical studies, trials and reviews exploring the potential use of herbs in the management of a huge array of disease, particularly cancer. But when exploring the evidence around the efficacy of such herbs, we need to change the lens through which we understand them and the uniquely synergistic ways in which herbs work in the face of cancer. This is because herbs are not chemically engineered pharmaceutical medicines, nor do they work in the same way as them.

When the pharmaceutical industry creates a new drug, it will typically identify a whole herb that shows promise in treating a particular health issue and then isolate the specific compound that is responsible for this action. It will then find ways to concentrate this compound to increase its bioavailability in the body so that it works more powerfully and effectively. As a singular example of this process, researchers undertook studies to explore what plants traditional herbalists used to treat heart disease. One exciting herb to emerge from this exploration was the common foxglove plant, which grows extensively across Western Europe. Traditional healers, particularly in France, have used this herb to treat heart failure, congestive artery disease and arrhythmias for centuries. Upon detailed investigation, these benefits were attributed to the cardiac glycosides found within foxgloves, which were subsequently isolated and developed into the licensed pharmaceutical drug digoxin – one of the most widely prescribed heart drugs in the world.

The process of isolating, removing and concentrating individual plant-based compounds in this way is not necessarily a bad thing; the synthetic drugs that such a process creates save countless lives every year. However, this is not how herbal medicines work. Herbs are incredibly complex in design and any given herbal medicine will typically contain hundreds of individual bioactive compounds that account for its healing capacity. And within the natural world, there are no spare parts. If a herb contains ninety-six individual plant-based compounds, all of those compounds, to a greater or lesser extent, are essential for harnessing the full healing potential of that plant. As soon as we extract a particularly important compound and ignore all the others, we immediately lose the synergistic and unique healing potential of that herb.

A great example of this is arguably the most famous Ayurvedic anti-cancer herb of them all: turmeric. In the Western clinical understanding, it is an isolated compound found within turmeric called curcumin that is said to be responsible for the potent anti-cancer actions observed in the

## Using Herbal Medicines Safely

In the face of cancer, everyone's body, immune status, liver functionality and myriad other physiological variables are different. When deciding to use these herbs, the most important consideration before all others is to ensure that it is safe for you to do so. The best way to ensure this is to maintain complete transparency with your consultant and clinical care team. Organise to meet with them and tell them that you are thinking about starting an evidence-based herbal medicine regime as a supportive therapy to your conventional cancer care. Tell them the specific herbal medicines you are looking to start and your rationale for doing so. And to allow your consultant to make an informed decision about your request, signpost them to an incredibly helpful online resource managed by one of the world's leading cancer research centres, the Memorial Sloan Kettering Cancer Center (MSKCC) in the US. The MSKCC leads the way in the integrative management of cancer that combines the very best of both conventional and complementary medicine. To support this objective, they run an exceptionally well-researched and up-to-date herbal medicine database, which can be found at www.mskcc.org/cancer-care/diagnosis-treatment/symptom-management/integrative-medicine/herbs/search. This database provides detailed and evidence-based explorations of all the primary herbal medicines used in cancer care and has sections for patients and for healthcare professionals. All the herbal medicines discussed in this chapter are included and, crucially, all of the potential side effects, safety issues and herb–drug interactions are clearly listed. Providing your consultant with access to this database will allow them to assess the safety and merits of using the herbs covered in this chapter in your unique clinical circumstances. If, and only if, your consultant is happy for you to use the herbal formulation described in Using These

> Herbs on page 134, then you can do so with the confidence that your clinical care team are fully aware of this and have deemed it safe. This greatly reduces the risk of any adverse reactions or negative herb–drug interactions. However, if your consultant is of the opinion that these herbs are not safe for you to use, please follow their advice as they are best placed to make this decision based upon their in-depth knowledge of your clinical status.

clinical research. However, curcumin accounts for less than 5 per cent of the bioactivity found within turmeric root, which contains more than three hundred additional bioactive constituent parts. But these additional three hundred compounds are vital to activating the anti-cancer activity of curcumin. So much so that when curcumin has been tested in clinical studies in isolation, it consistently underperforms in comparison to when turmeric is used as a whole herb that contains all of its constituent parts, including curcumin. For example, researchers have observed that compared to isolated curcumin, whole turmeric was able to impart significantly greater impact upon regulating inflammatory markers, blood sugar levels and cell division control.[3] Given that all three of these variables are physiologically implicated in cancer biology, this is valuable research.

A similar study that is equally important for us to consider in the context of cancer survivorship is the impact of whole turmeric versus isolated curcumin on the expression of a protein called perforin. Perforin plays an integral role in the regulation of immune activity, including immune activity in the tumour microenvironment. It is also instrumental in the regulation of cell replication and thus is a key regulatory mechanism relevant to cancer cell proliferation. Crucially, researchers observed that whole turmeric, in its pure and unadulterated form, significantly outperformed isolated curcumin in the positive regulation of perforin.[4] It is clear to see that the observable anti-cancer benefits of pure, whole turmeric are significantly greater than the concentrated use of its specific parts.

While this is a single example of one particular herb, the same principle applies to all herbs in all contexts. Herbs are beautifully intricate, intelligent and bioactive entities that are able to induce profound changes in the physiological workings of the body. When we are using herbs, we need to recognise the truly unique holism within plant medicines and use this to fuel a reverence for the way we understand and use herbs. Doing so asks us to respect the latent power inherent in whole herbs while also being fully mindful of the evidence that highlights just how clinically active they are in their anti-cancer capacity. With the explosion of new health supplements entering the market that are derived from isolated herbal compounds as opposed to whole herbs, this book instead endorses the use of pure and unadulterated herbs. Using herbs in this way ensures we stay true to the authentic practices of traditional systems of medicine such as Ayurveda while also affording us greater clinical efficacy, as the turmeric example so clearly highlights.

There is also another primary benefit of only using whole herbs in this way: better safety profiles. When you isolate an individual compound from a herb and package this into a supplement, you create an incredibly potent product that contains levels of phytonutrients in massively greater concentrations than nature intended. These isolated and concentrated herbal supplements, being in an unnatural form, are far more likely to cause side effects and adverse reactions in comparison to using whole herb equivalents in their natural form as gifted to us by nature.

When used properly, herbal medicines can be of immense value within the overarching arena of cancer survivorship. Using herbal medicines in this way has been shown to be one of the nine most common practices adopted by those going on to experience exceptional cancer survivorship, particularly in those with advanced and incurable cancers.[5] The sections in this chapter provide a detailed and evidence-based exploration of a selection of the most important anti-cancer herbs and how best to use them in a safe and effective way.

## The Anti-Cancer Herbal Pharmacy

There are hundreds of herbal medicines from around the world that possess proven anti-cancer activity. When we refer to anti-cancer activity in this way, it specifically means the ability of any given herb to help suppress the growth and proliferation of cancer cells via a multitude of mechanisms. That might be the activation of immune activity within the tumour microenvironment, the stimulation of death in cancer cells or the suppression of cancer cell proliferation. Thus, the hallmarks of cancer suppression that we applied as the framework for understanding anti-cancer nutrition in chapter 5 also apply here. You will remember that these hallmarks were a systematically developed framework for understanding the primary mechanisms that cancer uses to evade destruction and promote continual growth. And as we shall see below, all of the discussed herbs we will explore have published clinical evidence to show their efficacy in suppressing one or more of these primary hallmarks of cancer. Given the sheer volume of herbal medicines from around the world that fulfil this criterion, it was very difficult to decide upon which herbs to focus on here. And because a full treatise on the world's collective formulary of anti-cancer medicinal herbs is beyond the scope of this book, I made my selection based on the criteria that the herbs:

- are easy to source and obtain
- have robust evidence to support their use
- have clear data to show when they are safe to use and, more importantly, when they aren't
- are most celebrated within the Ayurvedic framework in relation to cancer survivorship

I have narrowed this choice down to five Ayurvedic medicinal herbs that, safety permitting, can be combined into one single herbal prescription to be used daily. So, before we discuss how to adopt herbal medicines into our daily self-care routine, let us first explore these five primary Ayurvedic anti-cancer herbs in more detail.

## *Amla*

**Alternative Names** Common name: Indian gooseberry. Latin: *Emblica officinalis*. Sanskrit: *Amalaki*.

### Overview
From the Sanskrit, amalaki translates as 'the fruit in which dwells the goddess of prosperity', highlighting the view that those who consume this herb become endowed with prosperity in their spiritual, material and physical lives, including their health status. More commonly known as amla or the Indian gooseberry, it is one of the most valued and worshipped plants in Ayurveda, from both a medicinal and spiritual perspective, whose use goes

back thousands of years. In the *Charaka Samhita*, which is thought to have been composed as early as 400 BCE, it is stated that of all the rejuvenating and strengthening tonic herbs in Ayurveda, amla is to be considered the most important, effective and powerful. There is much Western evidence to support this claim, not least that amla is officially regarded as being the highest natural source of vitamin C found anywhere in the plant kingdom; one fruit (the size of a small grape) contains more vitamin C than three to four oranges!

## Botanical and Phytochemical Make-up

Amla is a small gooseberry-sized fruit that grows on the *Emblica officinalis* tree, which is indigenous to both tropical and subtropical regions of India and the Middle East. Aside from possessing massive levels of vitamin C, the amla berry also contains a variety of vital phytonutrients such as phenolic acids, flavonoids, tannins and other phenolics, along with calcium, potassium, iron and B-vitamins.[6]

## Evidence Overview

In ovarian cancer cells, amla has been shown to possess metastases-inhibiting impacts by suppressing the ability of cells to invade neighbouring tissues.[7] In the same study, amla was also shown to inhibit angiogenesis, the process that tumours use to pull in new blood vessels to fuel growth. Similarly, and crucially, amla was shown to suppress a key cancer growth promoter called IGF-1 (insulin-like growth-factor 1), which has been linked to better outcomes in many cancers.[8] The massive volume of plant-based polyphenols found in amla have been shown to help protect against DNA damage, regulate cancer-specific inflammatory mechanisms and promote cancer cell cycle arrest in many different types of cancer.[9] Additionally, there is mounting evidence that amla can help protect against the side effects and toxicity of both radiotherapy and chemotherapy.[10] Test tube studies have also revealed that amla is clinically effective in killing a wide variety of different cancer cells, including lung, ovarian, cervical and breast cancers.[11] Finally, amla is a potent immune stimulant that can help to optimise the overall functionality of the immune system, largely due to the massive levels of antioxidants found within the berry.[12] And while it is important to highlight that much of the above research has been conducted primarily in laboratory and rodent studies, it provides a strong rationale for why this potent anti-cancer herbal medicine is so valued and so revered within the Ayurvedic framework.

## 2. Ashwagandha

**Alternative Names** Common name: Winter cherry. Latin: *Withania somnifera-Radix*. Sanskrit: *Asva-gandha*.

### Overview

As one of the most important herbal medicines in Ayurveda, ashwagandha has been used in India for thousands of years, with the first medicinal writings on it appearing around six thousand years ago. So famous was this herb that Alexander the Great reportedly gave it to his armies before battle to empower them with greater strength, energy and stamina. In Sanskrit, the name ashwagandha translates as the 'smell of a horse', which has a twofold meaning. Firstly, when ground up, ashwagandha smells slightly horsey and earthy. More important, however, is its second metaphorical meaning: the regular consumption of ashwagandha is said to impart the strength, stamina and vitality of a pureblood stallion.

### Botanical and Phytochemical Make-Up

Ashwagandha is a small, nondescript shrub that prefers the relatively arid and sandy soils of more temperate regions of India and Sri Lanka. It is typically quite a small plant, growing to only around two feet in height. While all parts of the plant reportedly have medicinal value, it is the roots that are most commonly used as medicine. These roots contain a myriad of medically active compounds including the celebrated withanalides, which are responsible for many of the healing impacts attributed to ashwagandha. The roots also contain a treasure trove of other powerful compounds including massive levels of antioxidants, among them superoxide and glutathione (which possess proven anti-cancer actions), iron, amino acids, choline, alkaloids and anti-cancer lignans and tannins.

### Evidence Overview

Ashwagandha has been employed as an anti-cancer herb within the framework of Ayurveda for millennia. And much modern-day clinical research supports this notion, showing that ashwagandha, and the compounds it contains, are active against many of the primary hallmarks of cancer previously discussed. For example, research has observed that ashwagandha can help block cancer cell proliferation, reactivate the activity of tumour suppressor genes, suppress angiogenesis, inhibit metastatic progression, stabilise the genome, suppress pro-cancer anti-inflammatory pathways and improve cancer-specific immune activity.[13] Of additional interest is that the use of ashwagandha has been shown to reduce chemotherapy-induced neutropenia.[14] And while this research was conducted in mice, it provides early evidence for the use of herbs such as ashwagandha alongside chemotherapy to help reduce treatment side effects. Similarly, in those with breast cancer, the use of ashwagandha was shown to alleviate chemotherapy-induced fatigue and improve quality of life.[15]

## 3. Astragalus

**Alternative Names** Common name: milk-vetch root. Latin: *Astragalus membranaceua*.

### Overview

Astragalus originates in China, where it is revered as one of the most important of all herbal medicines. Within Traditional Chinese Medicine (TCM), astragalus is known as *huang qi*, meaning 'yellow leader'. This name refers to the deeply yellow coloured interior of the root but more so to the plant's position of prestige among Chinese medicine practitioners, who often refer to it as the 'leader of all other herbal medicines'. Over the last few decades, this incredible herb has been powerfully adopted not only into the Ayurvedic framework of herbalism but also into the Western arena of evidence-based herbal research due to the profound health benefits it has been shown to afford. This is particularly true in the context of immune health and the alleviation of many of the common side effects of conventional cancer treatments, as explored below.

### Botanical and Phytochemical Make-up

Astragalus is a herbaceous perennial, growing to around twenty-five to forty centimetres in height. It grows in grassy regions and on mountainsides, requiring plenty of exposure to the sun. The roots are dried and then sliced for distribution. The slices are yellow in colour and have a sweet, moistening taste with a firm, fibrous texture. Contained with the herb are a selection of powerful constituents such as triterpenoid saponins, polysaccharides, isoflavonoids, phytosterols and essential oils. It is these (both individually and collectively), that are responsible for the health gains associated with the use of astragalus.

### Evidence Overview

Due to its traditional use as an anti-cancer herb, astragalus has attracted much clinical research attention over the last two decades. Across the board, this foundation of research has shown astragalus to possess potent anti-cancer actions in a wide variety of contexts. For example, clinical research has shown astragalus to exhibit anti-cancer activity against lymphomas and colorectal, ovarian, stomach, liver, lung, cervical, breast and nasopharyngeal cancer.[16] It has been shown to induce aggressive apoptosis (cell death) in many types of cancer lines while also inhibiting the process of angiogenesis and tissue invasion.[17] Similarly, astragalus has potent immune-modulating impacts and has been shown to positively alter anti-cancer immune activity specifically within the tumour microenvironment.[18] It is probably due to a combination of these mechanisms that astragalus has been associated with prolonged survival times in certain types of cancer such as acute myeloid leukaemia.[19] Furthermore, astragalus has been shown to significantly reduce the side effects of both chemotherapy and radiotherapy treatments,[20] including the reversal of chemotherapy-induced immune-suppression.[21] Yet more research highlights report a reduction in chemotherapy-induced nausea and vomiting,[22] reduced fatigue[23] and improvements in overall quality of life.[24]

## 4. Triphala

### Overview

Triphala is without doubt the most famous herbal formulation within the Ayurvedic framework. As a formulation, it is not a single herb but is rather made up of equal parts of three dried super-fruits, amla (*Emblica officinalis*), bhibitaki (*Terminalia bellirica*) and haritaki (*Terminalia chebula*). Each of these three herbs is incredibly powerful in its own right, but by combining them together the whole becomes significantly greater than the sum of their parts. Interestingly, Charaka, who composed the *Charaka Samhita* and is arguably the most famous Ayurvedic physician of all, regarded triphala as one of the most important and effective Ayurvedic medicines. Charaka is said to have personally foraged and prepared the highest quality triphala for the King of Kushan (now known as Kashmir) in the first century CE to help optimise his strength and vitality; this obviously worked as historical records show that the king lived to the age of 102, which is a remarkable achievement in that era.

## Botanical and Phytochemical Make-up

As a combination of three dried super-fruits, Triphala possesses an abundance and broad variety of phytonutrients. Specifically, it contains massive levels of antioxidants that originate from the flavonoids, polyphenols, saponins and high volumes of vitamin C contained within the fruit. It also possesses high concentrations of three further antioxidants – gallic acid, ellagic acid and chebulinic acid – all of which have been shown to possess anti-cancer actions.

## Evidence Overview

The clinical investigation of triphala has observed that it possesses anti-proliferative and apoptosis-inducing properties in a variety of cancers, including breast and prostate cancer.[25] It has also been shown to slow the growth rates and migration capacity of human gastric cancer cells.[26] A unique action that has been shown to be initiated by triphala is its ability to potentially modulate the p53 gene.[27] As we learned in the section Evading Growth Inhibitors on page 69 in chapter 5, clinical evidence shows that it is very difficult for a healthy cell to become cancerous unless it deactivates p53 genetic activity, but most cancers have evolved to achieve this. Early research suggests that triphala may offer potential in the reactivation of genetic cancer-suppressing mechanisms, although further research is required. Additionally, the high antioxidant levels found in triphala have been shown to activate a particularly potent antioxidant called ROS (reactive oxygen species). ROS has been shown to possess anti-cancer actions and specifically in triphala it was shown to induce cell death in breast cancer cells.[28] Another key research highlight is that triphala has been shown to suppress the activity of the inflammatory compound nuclear factor-kappa B (NF-κB), which fuels the growth of cancer cells. Virtually every action that cancer cells use to promote their own survival is supported by the role of NF-κB and triphala's potential to suppress this mechanism may, in part, explain its anti-cancer actions.[29] Lastly, triphala possesses important and proven immune-modulatory benefits, both generally and specifically within the tumour microenvironment.[30]

## 5. Turmeric

**Alternative Names** Common name: Turmeric. Latin: *Curcuma longa*. Sanskrit: *Haridra*.

### Overview

Turmeric is one of the most prized and revered herbs within Ayurveda and is commonly referred to by its colloquial name of *jayanti*, which translates from the Sanskrit as 'the one that is victorious over disease'. This is an apt title as turmeric is one of the most significant and clinically investigated herbal medicines in the world, showing efficacy in the management and prevention of a whole raft of diseases. Turmeric is also very much the celebrity of the anti-cancer herbal medicine research, with decades of evidence to highlight its efficacy in the suppression of cancer cell biology, as explored below.

### Botanical and Phytochemical Make-up

Turmeric is a perennial rhizome (an underground stem much like a root) that grows abundantly across India and Sri Lanka. Peeling the fresh rhizome reveals an explosion of orange/yellow, which is made by the yellow pigment in curcumin, one of the most active compounds found within turmeric. Found within the rhizome is an abundance and complex array of phytonutrients that are responsible for its health-giving abilities. These include essential oils, such as sesquiterpene bisabolenes, zingiberene, phellandrene, sabinene, cineole and borneol, as well as terpenes and curcuminoids such as curcumin.

### Evidence Overview

Extensive research over the last three decades has produced compelling evidence that turmeric, and the active compounds found within it, are able to evidentially interrupt multiple cell signalling pathways relevant to the suppression of cancer development, growth and progression.[31] This includes the promotion of apoptosis in cancer cells, the suppression of angiogenesis, the inhibition of cancer cell proliferation, blocking the mechanisms of tissue invasion and spread, the reduction of pro-cancer inflammatory mechanisms, high levels of antioxidant defence and the blocking of cancer-promoting NF-κB. (For a full overview of the anti-cancer actions of turmeric, see reference [32].) Turmeric has also shown efficacy in the alleviation of both chemotherapy- and radiotherapy-induced side effects, including reducing the levels of pain and inflammation experienced by those with breast cancer progressing through chemotherapy treatments.[33] Currently, clinical trials are underway to ascertain the impacts of turmeric as a supportive therapy in the management of blood cancers such as multiple myeloma.[34] However, there is clear evidence to suggest that turmeric can negatively interact with certain types of chemotherapeutic drugs, so it is absolutely essential that you check with your clinical care team before using this herb in any capacity.

## Using These Herbs

We now need to explore how best to use these five evidence-based herbal medicines. However, before we do so, a small caveat is needed: when using herbal medicines in the context of cancer survivorship, personalised advice and care can make all the difference. I strongly recommend that you seek the advice of a qualified Ayurvedic clinician or medical herbalist so that they can support and advise you in an individualised and safe way. Similarly – and this is imperative – please read the Using Herbal Medicines Safely section on page 124 before using any of the herbs discussed in this chapter, particularly if you are currently undergoing any form of conventional cancer treatment.

With those important points covered, I would like to discuss a simple and easy way of integrating these herbs into your daily self-care regime. Doing so involves the use of a 'polyherbal formulation' – that is, a formulation made up of several different herbs into one prescription. The benefit of using a polyherbal formulation in this way is that it harnesses the power of herbal synergy. Herbal synergy is when the entire therapeutic impact of a herbal formulation is greater than the sum of its individual parts. This becomes possible by the subtle interactions that occur when different herbs are combined together, with each herb increasing the bioavailability and impact of the other herbs. The easiest way to harness all of the benefits of the above herbal medicines is to combine them into a single formulation. Doing so makes them quick and easy to use and maximises the therapeutic impact they afford. The following instructions provide full guidance on how to do so.

### AYURVEDIC ANTI-CANCER FORMULATION

**Step 1:** First, you need to source the herbs. When doing so, it is important that you only purchase herbs from certified and reputable companies that can guarantee the quality and safety standards of the herbs they supply – see Herbal Medicines in appendix 3 (page 227) for a selection of certified herbal suppliers. To start with, you will need to order:

- 100 grams ashwagandha powder
- 100 grams triphala powder
- 100 grams astragalus powder
- 100 grams turmeric powder
- 40–50 millilitres amla juice or 100 grams amla powder

**Step 2:** Once you have your herbs, the next step is to blend them. Add each of your dried herbs to a clean, dry mixing bowl; do not add the amla juice or powder at this point. Then slowly and methodically mix all the herbs together until they are fully combined.

**Step 3:** Decant your blended herb mix into a clean, dry glass jar (such as a large jam jar or, better still, a Kilner-style jar) and seal it with an airtight lid.

**Usage:** To use your herbal formulation, put 1 teaspoon of the herbal blend into a glass and add a good pinch of freshly ground black pepper. Then, if using fresh amla juice, pour this into the glass; if you are using amla powder, mix this with 40 to 50 millilitres of water and add this to the glass. Stir well and drink. Make and drink this each morning and evening around food.

## A Word on the Ayurvedic Kitchen Herbal Pharmacy

Before we conclude this chapter, I would like to explore one final aspect of herbal medicine that is as beautiful as it is effective and as easy to adopt as it is enjoyable. And that's the concept of the Ayurvedic kitchen herbal pharmacy, which in many ways sits right at the very heart of Ayurvedic living. The Ayurvedic kitchen herbal pharmacy is based upon the traditional belief that in the quest to optimise health, maximise longevity and treat disease, there is no discernible difference between the kitchen as a place to prepare nutritious food and the kitchen as a place to prepare herbal remedies, tonics and medicines. For in the same way that we can add fennel seeds into a soup or casserole to add a rich depth of taste, that same fennel will also help to optimise our digestion, support our gut health and promote immune activity.[35] Or when making a beautifully aromatic mushroom curry, the use of medicinal mushrooms that possess proven anti-cancer actions, such as shiitake,[36] can turn our meal from a good one to a great one. The application of this model is infinite in scope but ultimately has one aim: to transform any meal you are making into a profoundly more healthy one with the broader and most concentrated use of culinary herbs. And when we approach this model specifically in the context of cancer, we are blessed by the fact that so many store cupboard herbs and spices can be pressed into service not just in the creation of delicious meals but also in terms of the proven anti-cancer actions they possess.

When constructing your meals, the liberal addition of a broad variety of culinary herbs is strongly advocated. This is because the majority of such herbs are concentrated phytonutrients powerhouses that can significantly optimise our overall health and immune status. Even more so, most herbs that lend themselves well to culinary use contain compounds that have been shown to possess proven anti-cancer actions, including potent antioxidant defence, the inhibition of pro-cancer inflammatory pathways, the deactivation of carcinogenic compounds, the suppression of several primary cancer promotion pathways (including the avoidance of apoptosis, the promotion of angiogenesis and the evasion of immune detection) and much else besides.[37] Generously adding such herbs to our cooking, seasoning and also herbal teas allows us to build up within our body an accumulative volume of the anti-cancer compounds. My top favourites here include:

| Rosemary | Cumin | Black nigella seeds |
| --- | --- | --- |
| Thyme | Fennel | Chilli |
| Sage | Black pepper | Cloves |
| Parsley | Ginger | Coriander (seeds |
| Basil | Turmeric | and leaves) |

Before we conclude this chapter, I would like to pay homage to one of the single best ways of integrating these kinds of culinary herbs into our daily life: authentic Ayurvedic chai. This classic tea dates back over five thousand years to when it was believed to have been created by the Ayurvedic physicians of the Royal Court of India as a tonic to build strength, energy and immunity, to suppress disease and promote ojas and longevity among members of the royal household. It also tastes divine. An added benefit is that the herbs and spices used within this classic chai all possess proven health benefits, particularly in the context of their specific anti-cancer actions.

So, after you finish reading this chapter, why not pop into your kitchen and spend a few minutes mindfully crafting this beautiful herbal infusion. And then, once it's ready to drink, perhaps sit down somewhere quietly and enjoy a blissful period of peaceful introspection, focusing on all the effort you are putting in to transforming your health and bringing your mind to bear on the fact that the path to exceptional is open to all of us, all of the time. Make this belief your reality and let it permeate every cell of your being until you feel, and experience in your very body, a powerful sense of optimism and excitement about your future.

**AUTHENTIC AYURVEDIC CHAI**

1½–2 cups water
6 black peppercorns, gently crushed
4 cardamom pods, gently crushed
3 cloves, gently crushed
1 teaspoon freshly grated ginger
2 cinnamon sticks
½–1 cup unsweetened almond milk
1 tablespoon loose-leaf black tea or 1 teabag (optional)
Raw honey, to taste

**Instructions**:
1. Place the water and all the herbs into a saucepan, bring to the boil and then simmer for 5–10 minutes. (The longer you leave it to simmer, the stronger the tonic becomes.)
2. Then, add the almond milk and simmer for another 1–2 minutes, stirring really well.
3. Turn off the heat. If you are using tea, add the tea leaves or teabag and leave to steep for a few minutes, depending on how strong you would like the tea to be.
4. Strain the infusion into a mug. Add some immune-boosting raw honey to taste – I like 1 teaspoon – and drink hot.

## Chapter Affirmations for My Journey to Becoming Exceptional

1. I consciously acknowledge the transformative power of the nature's pharmacy of herbal medicines and the evidence-based healing impacts they have on my body.

2. I endeavour to fully explore the application and integration of evidence-based herbal medicines as a vital component of my overall survivorship protocol.
3. I will do this in a safe and transparent way under the full guidance and support of my consultant and clinical care team.
4. If possible, I will seek the personalised advice of a qualified Ayurvedic clinician or medical herbalist for individualised herbal support.
5. **Summary Affirmation:** Each and every day, I will harness and unleash the full health-giving powers of the natural world's herbal pharmacy as I powerfully and purposefully progress along the path of becoming exceptional.

# CHAPTER EIGHT

# Dancing to Nature's Rhythm
## Chronobiology and the New Frontier of Cancer Survivorship

> *Light is life.*
> STEVEN MAGEE, *Hypoxia,*
> *Mental Ilness and Chronic Fatigue*

To study the workings of the natural world all around us is to observe a perfectly choreographed dance that moves to the infinite and soundless beat of nature's rhythms. This is a life-preserving dance that ensures the harmonious workings of every living thing on our planet. And if we have the eyes to see and the ears to hear, we can witness this dance playing out all around us; birds never forget to awaken and welcome each new day with their beautifully harmonised dawn chorus. Flowers never forget to effortlessly track the sun as it moves across the sky. Wild animals never forget that the setting of the sun each night is their cue to find shelter and fall into deep and restful sleep. The list goes on but the point remains; the entire natural world and everything in it has a perfectly orchestrated and intuitive knowledge of how to effortlessly follow and stay aligned with the rhythms of the natural world.

In Ayurveda, this intuitive knowledge is called *rta*, a concept that is as beautiful as it is powerful. Rta is the inner intelligence that exists as an inherent quality of every living thing and one that allows it to function and thrive in the most effective and harmonious way possible. And the concept of rta spans everything from the macrocosm to the microcosm. For example, at the macro level it is rta that keeps the planets of our solar system on their correct orbit around the sun. It is rta that keeps our earth spinning on its correct axis and it is rta that allows the moon to exert the correct gravitational pull upon the ocean's tides. At the micro level, rta allows our lungs to supply oxygen to our body and remove toxic carbon dioxide. It is rta that allows our cells to absorb nutrients and produce energy and rta that allows your eyes to see, your mind to comprehend and your heart to beat. To live in harmony with rta is to harmonise the entire workings of our body in such a way as to transform it. At the most fundamental level, the rta of every living thing on our planet has evolved to live in harmony with, and be optimally regulated by, the daily cycles of light and dark, day and night. In other words, to be harmoniously aligned with our planet's twenty-four-hour cycle. Indeed, scientific evidence now shows that this twenty-four-hour circadian cycle exerts the single biggest influence on how all organic matter functions and behaves, from giant mammals and minuscule birds to towering trees and tiny subterranean seeds.

It is because of their harmonious alignment with this twenty-four-hour circadian rhythm that birds will never forget to wake and sing their dawn chorus. Or why a flower will never fail to track the sun across the sky. It is impossible for them to not do so as the action is not consciously driven by them but rather by the all-pervading influence exerted by the sun. And, fortunately, there isn't one species on the planet that has the ability to override the all-pervading influence of this circadian cycle. In the wild, you would never find a diurnal (daytime-active) mammal hunting and feeding at night. It just never happens. Every single species effortlessly and intuitively follows their inbuilt circadian cycles and through doing so harnesses the full potential of rta. Every species except humans, that is. And the implications of our species' unique ability to consciously disconnect with our circadian rhythm represent arguably one of the biggest threats to our health and wellbeing that we are currently facing.

To fully grasp the significance of this threat, we have to remember that as a species we are evolutionarily speaking no different to a lion, polar bear or swallow. We originated in, evolved among and have spent the majority of our two-hundred-thousand-year history intimately linked to the natural world. Before the Stone Age revolution ten thousand years ago, we lived almost exclusively in hunter-gatherer communities. We, too, would have risen with the sun and gone to bed with its setting, we would only ever have eaten when it was light and slept when it was dark and we would never have engaged in complex mental tasks in the night because we would have been asleep, as nature intended. And through living in sync with our twenty-four-hour circadian cycle in this way, we would have helped to ensure the harmonious and optically balanced physiological health and functioning of our body.

But then disaster struck. As we progressed as a species, we found ways to override our inbuilt circadian rhythm. For example, we invented candles and then light bulbs that allowed us to work after dark and TVs that stimulate our minds when we should be sleeping, which can negatively affect our hormonal and immune status. We have access to food twenty-four hours a day and yet we are governed by our circadian clock to only eat in sunlight hours. This has resulted in longer periods of food intake that has spawned the explosion of metabolic problems such as elevated blood sugar, insulin resistance and obesity, all of which are implicated in the context of cancer.[38] We have twenty-four-hour gyms that allow us to exercise late at night when the physiology of the body is primed for restful sleep, not physical exertion, which can lead to compromised immune status and increased risks of infection. And underpinning it all, we live in a twenty-four-hour industrialised society that values productivity, longer working hours and relentless mental and physical activity over the honouring of our inbuilt and immutable waking, eating and sleeping circadian cycles. These types of misaligned societal, lifestyle and behavioural patterns have heralded the advent of one of the most destructive changes in human physiology in the history of our species: circadian disruption.

Circadian disruption is the title given to the all-pervasive and incredibly damaging physiological conditions that arise in the body when we live in a way that isn't in harmony with our inbuilt and genetically governed circadian clock. And as we shall see as we progress through this chapter, there isn't one cell in our body – not one – that isn't directly impacted upon and regulated by our circadian clock.[39] Thus, if we are to experience a move into optimal health and fully mobilise our healing potential, it is imperative that we learn to shift our daily rhythms in a way that ensures that our primary behaviours – when we wake, eat, work, sleep and exercise – are fully aligned with our circadian clock. Doing so has profoundly positive impacts upon a whole raft of health variables including the optimisation of immune activity, reduced inflammation, improved digestive and metabolic function, more effective DNA repair, optimal gene expression, improved mood and much else besides.[40] So important is the role of circadian alignment that it has spawned a whole new field of scientific study called circadian medicine. This new field has been so impactful that in 2017 it won the Nobel Prize for medicine and physiology, which represents the world's most prestigious award for medical research.[41]

In the specific context of cancer, circadian medicine is opening up new frontiers and potentially paradigm-changing understandings of cancer cell biology. For example, evidence shows that circadian disruption can activate a whole raft of genetic and physiological actions that are implicated in the development, growth and progression of cancer [42]. Research has observed that circadian disruption represents an inherent trait in the majority of cancer cells and that the re-establishment of circadian alignment in cancer cells themselves can help slow down, and in some cases help to inhibit, cancer development and progression.[43] Furthermore, activating circadian alignment has been shown to induce powerful and clinically significant improvements in anti-cancer immune activity and a reduction in pro-cancer inflammatory status [44].

Learning how to restructure our lifestyle to ensure we enjoy a harmonious relationship with our inbuilt circadian rhythm is absolutely vital. On this point, both cutting-edge Western clinical research and the ancient wisdom traditions of Ayurveda are in complete agreement. Ayurveda possesses a whole clinical discipline devoted to the entrainment of our lives with our circadian clock called dinacharya, which we will explore further in the section Dinacharya on page 146. The aim of this chapter is to provide an evidence-based framework for allowing us to simply and effortlessly live in alignment with our circadian clock. And to do that, we firstly need to understand a little more about what our circadian rhythm actually is and, more specifically, why our waking times and exposure to early morning sunlight are so important in the collective regulation of our circadian mechanisms over each twenty-four-hour period.

## What Is the Circadian Rhythm?

I think it is fair to say that most people have probably had periods in their lives when they are acutely aware of how impactful their circadian rhythm is upon their sense of wellbeing. If you have ever been on a long-haul flight, then the almost inevitable fatigue, sleep disruption and constipation that you experience upon arriving at your destination are all a direct byproduct of disrupted circadian cycles. If you have ever worked late into the night and then found it impossible to get to sleep, or eaten food at unusual times and experienced digestive discomfort, or slept in late and felt tired and sluggish for the rest of the day, these signs and symptoms are all directly induced by circadian rhythm disruption. But what exactly is our circadian rhythm and why does it impact upon us in such a profound and all-pervading way?

To answer that question, we firstly need to travel deep into the brain to visit the body's neurological timekeeper, the hypothalamus. The almond-sized hypothalamus sits right at the very centre of the brain, where it performs its central role of regulating homeostasis in the body. You'll remember from our previous discussions that homeostasis is when the body is operating from a place of optimal physiological balance and function, which is the prerequisite for the cultivation of optimal health and healing. Because the hypothalamus is responsible for the regulation of homeostasis, it is in turn indirectly responsible for regulating every system of the body. Control and regulation of our hormone secretions, body temperature, digestion and metabolism, blood pressure, heart rate and myriad other variables are all governed by the strings being pulled by the hypothalamus.

To effectively perform this almost unimaginably complex role, the hypothalamus is dependent upon the cues and messages it receives from the systems of the body. When you feel hot, your hypothalamus induces sweating to cool you down. When you haven't eaten, your hypothalamus makes you feel hungry so that you eat. When you haven't slept, your hypothalamus makes you feel tired so that you rest, and so on. This two-way channel of communication is vital for the perseveration and optimisation of the physiological workings of the body. However, these cues are of secondary importance in comparison to the single biggest influencer on the workings of the hypothalamus: the presence of sunlight. Because within the hypothalamus sits one of the most significant and important physiological regulators to be found anywhere in the brain, the suprachiasmatic nucleus (SCN).

The SCN's sole task is to notice and respond to the presence of light (or its absence as observed during the night) and regulate the workings of the body accordingly. When you awaken each morning, the beautiful dawn light that you see streaming in through your bedroom window hits the retina of your eye, which instantly signals to the SCN that it is the start of a new day. The SCN then kicks in to activate and stimulate all of the myriad physiological changes in the body that must occur during daylight hours (as opposed to nighttime hours) to maintain optimal health and physiological function. For example, cortisol is released to fire up the body in preparation for the day ahead, digestive and metabolic activity is stimulated in preparation for eating, diurnal immune status is modulated to provide optimal immune protection over the coming day and hormone secretion is regulated in such a way as to support optimal daytime physiological regulation. Put simply, the presence of early morning light is the signal for your SCN to induce all of the changes your body needs to perform optimally until it is dark again.

Once the sun sets and darkness falls, the opposite happens. The presence of darkness (more correctly, the absence of light) tells your SCN that it is now nighttime and that the day is ending. As evolutionary diurnal (daytime-active) mammals, this is our neurological cue to 'switch off' the activity of all the daytime functions and 'switch on' the activity of our nighttime functions. Doing so helps ensure deep and restful sleep via the secretion of melatonin and all the essential physiological activities that occur almost exclusively during the hours of darkness, such as repairing physiological damage incurred over the previous day, the regulation of nocturnal immune status and the removal of toxins. And then, when dawn breaks the next morning, the whole twenty-four-hour cycle starts again. We can think of the SCN as our body's timekeeper that ensures every single one of the trillions of cells in the body, and the unique physiological functions they control, work in the right way and at the right time to ensure the maintenance of optimal health and the prevention (and management) of disease.

However, the SCN in the brain is not the only timekeeper operating in the body. Each and every one of our fifty-plus trillion cells also contains its own unique inner clock that is also calibrated to a twenty-four-hour cycle. These intercellular timekeepers are called 'periphery clocks'. Thus, we have an overarching 'master' clock in the brain that is controlled by the SCN, and we have individual clocks in each and every one of our cells. When our master clock and our individual cellular clocks are working in harmony with each other, we enter into the hallowed state of circadian alignment, which ensures that every cell of the body and the organ systems they inhabit are working in the correct way, and performing their correct functions, at the correct times. The implications of this in the context of cancer survivorship are profound because of the clinical evidence highlighting the vital interplay between proper circadian alignment and the control and activation of a whole raft of cancer-preventing and cancer-controlling mechanisms.[45]

For every other species on the planet, circadian alignment appears to be easy to maintain. However, as mentioned previously, humans have used their immensely powerful brains to engineer a world in which we can do what we want, when we want and how we want in a way that is in direct conflict with our circadian clocks. And this has made it very difficult for us to maintain circadian alignment. We are rarely exposed to early morning light due to disrupted waking times and curtained windows, which disrupts the SCN's regulation of our circadian clock over the next twenty-four hours. We also often eat at the wrong times, we are exposed to artificial light late into the evening, we work into the night and we go to bed too late. This abnormal circadian behaviour forces the clocks in our cells to set their own schedule based upon the stimulation they receive from our lifestyle choices and behaviours. Crucially, this means they are no longer taking their cue from the master clock in the brain, the SCN. And when our individual cell clocks start working in conflict with the master clock in our brain, it creates a state of circadian disruption.

This is the diametric opposite of circadian alignment and represents one of the most dangerous conditions we can find in the body. In fact, the physiological impacts of circadian disruption are so dangerous that the International Agency for Research on Cancer has classified it as a Group 2A human carcinogen due to the clear evidence highlighting the increased risks of cancer in those living with chronic circadian disruption.[46] For example, individuals who have experienced many years of shift work, and thus have lived with chronic circadian disruption, have been shown to experience significantly higher rates of many different types of cancer in comparison to population norms.[47] Furthermore, and of greater importance to those currently living with cancer, is the growing foundation of evidence linking circadian disruption to faster rates of cancer growth and spread and poorer survival times. For instance, early studies using mice with tumours revealed that those animals subjected to jetlag via the continual shifting of their light/dark cycle experienced significantly faster rates of tumour growth and poorer outcomes than those mice keeping to normal circadian cycles.[48] Another important study looked at the effects of circadian disruption on survival times in humans with brain cancer. Crucially, this study actually analysed the circadian regulation of the cancer cells themselves. The results revealed that those individuals with cancer cells that still possessed high levels of circadian alignment lived significantly longer than those whose cancer cells were not aligned in this way.

The mechanisms by which circadian regulation can so significantly impact upon cancer cell behaviour in this way is still not fully understood. However, what is known is that disrupted circadian signalling has been implicated in the activation of all of the primary physiological, immunological and metabolic mechanisms employed by cancer cells that allows them to fuel growth, evade immune destruction and invade distant parts of the body.[49] Viewed through this lens, we can very quickly see why the re-establishment of proper circadian alignment is of such importance in the specific context of cancer survivorship. To do so, we simply need to realign our lives and routines in such a way that ensures they are working with, rather than against, the immutable twenty-four-hour rhythm of the world in which we live. And to do that in the most organic and effortless way possible, we can turn to Ayurveda's sacred and all-encompassing blueprint of circadian medicine: dinacharya.

## Dinacharya: Ayurveda's Sacred Blueprint of Circadian Medicine

For me personally, the Ayurvedic science of dinacharya represents one of the most beautiful and important gifts that Ayurveda offers to the West. This is because its adoption empowers us with all of the knowledge we need to structure our days in such a way as to support proper and complete circadian alignment. But dinacharya also offers us a promise that is so much more than pure circadian alignment. It provides the branches from which we hang the transformative fruits of our daily self-care rituals. Dinacharya isn't just about 'time'. It is about what we do with that time.

So, while awakening at the correct time of the day is a vitally important aspect of circadian alignment from both an Ayurvedic and a Western perspective, dinacharya develops this further. If we can awaken at the right time *and* embed core self-care practices into this early morning period, such as meditation, Ayurvedic self-abhyanga massage (see page 152), reflective journalling and physical movement, we harness not only the full benefits of circadian alignment but also the transformative health benefits of the self-care practices we embed during this time. This allows us to start each new day in a way that has positively impacted upon the functioning of every cell in the body via re-establishing proper circadian control. But it also allows us to start each day having unleashed the benefits of a raft of self-care practices that have all been shown to impart important benefits in the context of immune function and cancer survivorship. And above and beyond these very important physiological benefits, following the blueprint of dinacharya also has an immeasurable impact upon our psychological and emotional wellbeing. It allows us to start each new day from a place of empowerment and autonomy. We have taken conscious action to inform our outlook, mindset and positivity over the next twenty-four hours. We spend the quiet and sacred hours of the morning acknowledging and awakening our infinite ability to be the architects of how each day unfolds in front of us in terms of our health, vitality, expectations, hopes, goals, aims, dreams and much more. In short, dinacharya gifts us with a time-tested blueprint for starting each precious new day in the very best possible way. And in receiving this gift, we are transformed by it.

## What Actually is Dinacharya?

From the Sanskrit, *dinacharya* is made from the root words *dina*, meaning 'day', and *acharya*, meaning 'activity' or 'rituals'. Thus, conceptually dinacharya translates as all the activities and rituals we embed each day to ensure we remain optimally aligned to the creative energy of the natural world. To do so, dinacharya asks us to synchronise our lives with the two primary energies present in each twenty-four-hour cycle: the solar energy and the lunar energy. As we have seen, it is the early morning solar energy that plays the single most important role upon the proper regulation of circadian alignment in the human body; the early morning represents the jumping-on point for harnessing the profound benefits of dinacharya. However, it is important to remember that to awaken early each morning revitalised and re-energised, it is imperative that we benefit from deep and rejuvenating sleep. Thus, while the solar cycle of day can, on the surface, seem to be more important than the lunar cycle of the night, this is misleading: the success of one is completely and wholly dependent upon the success of the other.

In the following sections, we will progress though a day perfectly lived as informed by a marriage of cutting-edge clinical circadian research alongside the timeless tradition of dinacharya. Before doing so, however, it is important to emphasise a key point. Our daily routines are as individual as we are and there will never be a one-size-fits-all blueprint that works for everyone. We need to ensure the daily routine we construct for ourselves fits into our lifestyle rather than forcing our lifestyle to fit the routine. It is counterproductive to persevere with a specific morning routine if doing so creates more stress, anxiety and conflict than it resolves. So be gentle on yourself in applying these principles. Take the routines that intuitively feel right for you and leave or modify the ones that don't. Remember, there is no wrong or right here, only wrong or right for you. If the routine outlined below would make your mornings too rushed because of the school run, delay it until you get home when you have the time and space to calmly enjoy it. Or if you have to leave the house very early each morning for work, perhaps try to embed the core practices in the evening.

The options are limitless but, in as much as it is possible for you, the following blueprint provides a structured framework for a day lived fully and perfectly aligned to nature's infinite intelligence. This blueprint focuses on three key elements: 1) waking times and the Ayurvedic optimal morning routine; 2) the importance of chrono-nutrition and eating times; and 3) the optimal evening routine to support deeply rejuvenating sleep. We will explore each of these stages in turn. And so we begin with the importance of harnessing the inherent power of *Brahma muhurta* and the Ayurvedic optimal morning routine.

## Brahma Muhurta: Ayurveda's Golden Hour and the Optimal Morning Routine

The first hour after sunrise stands alone and apart from any other time of the day. There is a unique energy to this time that is unmatched in its quality, impact and radiance, and a quietude that is almost palpable. The whole of the natural world is still largely at rest, and to stand outside is to experience a stillness that is beguiling. And yet, paradoxically, as the precious minutes of dawn tick away, this sense of stillness and quietude is replaced by an ever-increasing sense of awakening, energy and anticipation. As the sun rises higher in the eastern sky, and its intensity increases, the whole of the natural world comes alive as birds start to sing, flowers open and collective productivity of each and every species begins once again as another day commences: eating, moving and working.

To be awake at this time is to experience these same qualities in our own body and mind. As Ayurveda teaches us, 'As in the macrocosm, so in the microcosm'. By being receptively awake in the earlier part of the morning, we absorb and become the very stillness, peace and calmness present in the macrocosm. In my opinion, there is no better set of qualities to start the day with. But then, as the sun continues to rise and the morning advances, these qualities are slowly replaced by a growing sense of energy, vitality and physical awakening as our physiology fires up in preparation for the coming day.

In the Ayurvedic and Yogic traditions, this sacred time of the day is called Brahma muhurta, which translates from the Sanskrit as the 'creator's time' or 'sacred time'. Being awake, and in a contemplative and spiritually aligned state, during Brahma muhurta is of vital importance as it allows us to fully and completely calibrate the entire workings of our body and mind with the larger workings of the twenty-four-hour circadian cycle. In other words, it facilitates perfect circadian alignment.

What is fascinating is that the Ayurvedic interpretation of Brahma muhurta is in perfect harmony with the most advanced clinical research within the field of circadian medicine. Remember, it is the SCN within the hypothalamus that acts as the master clock in the brain. It keeps the collective functioning of the entire body, and every cell within it, in perfect circadian alignment over each twenty-four-hour cycle. Remember also that it is this early morning alignment that lays the foundation of health in every single cell in the body. Finally, remember that it is exposure to early morning light, such as that only experienced in Brahma muhurta, that acts as the primary mechanisms by which the SCN facilitates this process. So whether we view this fundamentally important concept through the lens of ancient Ayurvedic teachings or modern-day circadian biology, the conclusion is the same: to experience a move into optimal health requires the unleashing of the regulatory powers of proper circadian alignment that are only available to us in the early morning hours.

However, as previously mentioned, the Ayurvedic tradition moves this process along even further. Brahma muhurta is much more than simply waking at the correct time so as to ensure we expose our eyes to early morning sunlight. It is about harnessing the full power of the 'creator's time' by waking earlier and using this time to embed a transformative morning routine made up of a selection of self-care practices that go on to optimise the workings of the entire body.

This is called the Ayurvedic optimal morning routine. I have lived this morning routine for decades now and it is the cornerstone of my physical and mental wellbeing. It leaves me feeling motivated, engaged, vital, energised, optimistic, empowered and filled with health. And it induces these qualities *before* the day even begins. This then goes on to shape, and directly influence, how each day subsequently unfolds. I have taught this morning routine to thousands of people over the years, and I would say that, beyond perhaps anything else, it is the practice that has gone on to induce the single biggest positive change in physical, emotional and psychological health. To illustrate this, let us briefly explore the personal experiences of Liz and how she harnessed the power of Brahma muhurta to help transform every aspect of her life in the face of cancer.

## Liz's Experience of Brahma Muhurta

Liz was an otherwise healthy sixty-nine-year-old women who had been diagnosed with myeloma, an incurable form of blood cancer that affects our plasma cells, six months previously. This diagnosis had come completely out of the blue and had left Liz reeling. It had reawakened her propensity for anxiety, which she had suffered with all her life. She woke each morning with a sense of dread that persisted all through the day. She felt scared, disconnected and ungrounded.

During any quiet times of the day, she found herself continually catastrophising and thinking about the worst-case scenarios; how her cancer would progress, the incurability of her prognosis, the reality of her own mortality, anxiety about her beloved family and all the dreams and goals she would never get to realise. This mental turbulence left her feeling exhausted and she felt tired and physically drained most days. This then stopped her from doing lots of the things she loved, such as gardening and walking. Because she was moving less, the aches and pains in her knees and legs worsened.

As her mood dropped, she became less engaged in the world around her until one day she realised she needed to act to stop and reverse this rapid spiral of deterioration, which was quickly getting out of control. In her own words, her fear of dying was suffocating her passion for living. Liz came along to one of the eight-week cancer survivorship courses I was running at that time, a big emphasis of which was upon the importance of adopting Brahma muhurta. After the first session, she came to have a chat with me and explained her situation and said how much she needed a structured plan to help her escape the rut she found herself in. She confirmed with a fierce resolution to commit to adopting Brahma muhurta and the Ayurvedic optimal morning routine, starting the very next morning.

As the weeks unfolded, I would have regular chats with Liz after each session and sometimes over the phone too. And watching Brahma muhurta weave its magic into her life was an absolute privilege. She recounted how, even on the very first morning, just taking positive action to waken an hour earlier had a catalysing effect; she was proactively taking control of her situation rather than passively submitting to it. By spending quiet time in meditation each morning, she got a handle on her anxiety before it had a chance to build and she felt so much calmer as the day progressed. Rather than rushing headlong into her day, the one hour 'creator's time' gave her the opportunity to ease into it gently and to savour the peace and quiet of the early morning so that these same qualities could be reflected in her being.

The beautiful act of morning self-massage left her feeling supple and loose and reconnected her with her body; she no longer perceived her body as a diseased entity that had let her down but rather as a radiant temple that allowed her to fully and complete engage with the world and savour the rich tapestry of life to the fullest. By gently moving her body each and every morning with several rounds of Yogic sun salutations, her flexibility increased, her aches and pains lessened and her physical energy greatly improved. With this increased energy and confidence, she began to do more. She took up painting classes, planted her vegetable garden and rejoined her monthly walking circle. Because she was being, doing and living more, she felt a heavy but beautiful sense of tiredness each evening, which saw her going to bed earlier, sleeping better and waking earlier and more easily. In short, within eight short weeks she had turned her life around. Yes, there was still anxiety and there were still dark days. But the bad times never had the strength to overpower her any more.

She was in control of her situation, rather than her situation being in control of her. She was now the autonomous architect of how each day unfolded and, by winning her mornings, she won her days. And while Liz was doing much more besides Brahma muhurta to regain her sense of self, it was to her morning creator's time that she attributed her incredible turnaround.

## Embedding The Ayurvedic Optimal Morning Routine

Having discussed the concept of Brahma muhurta and the Ayurvedic optimal morning routine, we now need to look at exactly what it entails and how to practise it. The following provides a detailed guide for doing so. However, it is incredibly important to emphasise that the morning routine needs to be fluid, enjoyable and effortless; relinquish the need to practise the full routine perfectly every day and just enjoy what you can do on a day-by-day basis. One final point: try to commit to engaging with this morning routine, in whatever way works for you, for four weeks. In my experience of teaching this to people, if you can do this, by the time the four weeks are up, the improvements in physical and emotional health are so noticeable that it is very unlikely that you will ever stop engaging and practising it.

### 1. Waking Up

Classically speaking, there is lots of debate around the actual time of Brahma muhurta. However, from a practical perspective it is best to think of it as the period that spans the hour before and the first hour after sunrise. There is obviously a significant shift in this over the course of twelve months, with sunrise being much earlier in summer and much later in winter. To correct for this seasonal variation, a good blanket rule is to aim to wake no later than 6 am in the lighter summer months and no later than 7 am in the winter months. Doing so will ensure you are harnessing the early morning sunlight that is so important in relation to proper circadian alignment. Waking earlier will also give you extra time (ideally thirty to sixty minutes) to embed the practices inherent to the optimal morning routine. Depending upon when you currently wake up, a progressive approach to this is often helpful; aim to awaken fifteen minutes earlier every week until you reach the optimal time. This helps prevent any fatigue that can occur if you drastically alter your waking time very quickly. It is also important to emphasise that we are talking about *waking up* as opposed to *getting up*. Waking up at 6 am, making a cup of tea and heading back to bed to read or slowly come to is absolutely fine!

**Important Point:** If you are currently going through active cancer treatments and are suffering from noticeable fatigue or exhaustion, waking up earlier in this way is not always advisable; in these instances, the body needs more sleep and rest, and sleeping in later is beneficial. Thus, listen to your body and do what feels right.

## 2. Ayurvedic Oil Massage: Self-Abhyanga

Once you feel ready to get out of bed, the first practice is best performed in your bathroom as it involves a mindfully performed self-massage. Daily morning Ayurvedic oil massage is one of the most powerful rejuvenation regimes that you can add to your daily routine. The motion and pressure of the massage creates heat and friction on the skin, which helps to stimulate immunity, reduce inflammation, loosen up impurities, improve circulation, increase the health and vitality of the skin, and enliven the energy systems of the body.[50] Furthermore, daily self-massage can also induce profound gains upon our emotional and mental wellbeing. The skin is the single biggest regulator of our hormones and gently massaging the body every morning can help to balance and optimise our hormone profile.[51] This results in an increased secretion of our mood-boosting 'feel-good' hormones such as dopamine and serotonin while also helping to reduce our stress hormones. And the power of daily self-massage is that by practising it in the morning we have acted to balance and optimise our biochemistry *before* the day has even begun. Ayurvedic oil massage is especially good in the management of ailments such as weakness, stress, anxiety and fatigue. Most people report feeling much stronger, happier, more contented and more emotionally balanced throughout the day as a result of their morning self-massage.

Performing a self-massage is incredibly easy and the best bit is that we only need to practise it for four to five minutes to obtain all of these wonderful benefits. To perform your self-massage, take a small amount of hand-warm sesame oil and gently rub this over your whole body. Then, using slow rhythmic strokes, massage your right foot, right lower leg and right upper leg; it is helpful to use long flowing strokes over your long bones and round circular strokes on your joints. Then repeat on your left leg. Then gently massage your tummy using clockwise strokes before moving to your right hand, right lower arm and right upper arm. Repeat on your left arm. Then massage both shoulders (spend more time here as this is where we hold lots of tension), your neck and face, and try to be present and mindful during these sacred five minutes. It is best to perform the self-massage before you shower. Once finished, simply step into your shower or bath and wash your body as usual.

## 3. Self-Developing Practices – Meditation, Journalling and Prayer

Once you have performed your self-massage and showered, you should feel nicely awakened and invigorated. Now is the perfect time to embed a selection of practices that help to create an elevated state of calm, peace, empowerment, optimism and personal development. Great options here include meditation, journalling and/or prayer. We'll explore these in turn:

### i. Meditation

In chapters 3 and 4 we discussed in detail why practices like meditation and visualisation are of such importance within the field of cancer survivorship, and now is the perfect time to embed these practices. If you are new to meditation and visualisation, then you can use the free guided meditation links in chapter 3 to get you started. (See Practice 1 and Practice 2 on page 43.) Alternatively, there are some excellent meditation resources available online. My top recommendations include Headspace (www.headspace.com), Insight Timer (www.insighttimer.com) and Calm (www.calm.com).

If you already have an established meditation practice that works for you, then simply continue to use this. Ideally, try to meditate for at least twenty minutes during your morning routine.

## ii. Journalling

Journalling is a profoundly powerful self-care practice to start the day with and one that can discernibly impact how we engage with, and experience, the subsequent day. When describing the practice of morning journalling to those I work with, I always say that it is the single best practice for 'setting each new day up for greatness'. Spending five to ten minutes each morning writing in your journal can positively and directly impact how you want the upcoming day to unfold. For example, what kind of mindset do you want to foster today? What things are you most grateful for or looking forward to? What things are you worried, anxious or ruminating about right now? What things do you need to do today to make this day brilliant? When and where are you scheduling time for yourself, your hobbies, passions, friends, exercise and other important pursuits? What things didn't work so well yesterday that you want to improve upon today, such as eating a little better, exercising more, being more present with your loved ones or prioritising your self-care a little more? Writing in your journal in this way each morning about how you want to be, feel and act to make this coming day the best it can possibly be results in a tangible reflection of these qualities in our actual outer reality. While there are an infinite number of ways of using a journal, the following is the approach that I find most helpful.

### GRATITUDE

Starting the day with a gratitude practice has been proven to make us feel happier, more positive and less stressed.[52] The very first thing I write each morning in my journal is five things I am grateful for or looking forward to today. Doing so makes me more mindfully aware of all the amazing things in my life and helps keep my mind on what's good rather than what's not.

### HONEST REFLECTION

The next practice is to spend a little time reflecting on how you are feeling in your mind and body right now. How's your energy, mood and outlook? What's making life great right now and what's making it difficult? What is causing you the most stress or anxiety? How are your relationships with those you love the most? This practice is important because it increases our awareness of how we are in ourselves. And with increased awareness we can make better choices. And with better choices we almost always get better results. For example, imagine that this time of inner reflection flags up that you are feeling a little disconnected from a loved one because life is so busy right now and you haven't spent much quality time together recently. Increasing your awareness of this would allow you to schedule and prioritise a time this week for a lovely walk and picnic with this person, the result of which is that you rebuild that connection. Thus, a single aspect of daily life is improved simply by increased awareness. If we extrapolate this across our entire lives, it can't help but make it burn brighter.

#### FOCUS ON FIVE

The next practice is to list the five most important things that have to happen today to make this day brilliant. This covers the full spectrum of life: our work, family, hobbies, health, goals, dreams and much else besides. The aim being that when you review your day before drifting off to sleep (another great practice, by the way) you can honestly say to yourself that it was a day well lived. As I write this, I have my journal open next to me and I will share what my Focus on Five was for today: 1) ensuring the highest-quality writing I can possibly produce that will be of the greatest service to those living with cancer (today is a writing day); 2) move for two minutes after every hour of sitting to offset a more sedentary day; 3) be fully present with my attention this afternoon when I take my daughter horse riding; 4) prioritise a family meal tonight because we haven't had one for a few days; and 5) ensure every meal I eat today is saturated with goodness.

#### TO-DO LIST

Finally, I write a list of the more mundane things I have to do today. Getting these out of my head and onto paper frees up more mental space for important things and reduces any sense of overwhelm or anxiety.

So have a go at journalling in the sacred time of Brahma muhurta and experiment with it to see what works best for you. I would also advocate buying a journal just for this process and make it one that is aesthetically beautiful for you and one that you want to pick up, look at and write in. It sounds silly but you really do form a real emotional connection with your journal and it needs to be emotive in this capacity.

### iii. Prayer

Depending upon your spiritual or religious beliefs, this is a great time for prayer in whatever way that looks like for you. It could be the reading of sacred texts, chanting the rosary or simply 'saying your prayer' in the tradition of your practice.

## 4. Sun Salutations

Having woken at the correct time, self-massaged, showered and meditated, the emphasis of the morning now shifts from a more inward-looking contemplative focus to a more outward-looking dynamic focus. By this time, the sun should be climbing higher into the sky and the energy in the wider world all around us will be building. We need to replicate that building energy in the microcosm of our body. And the famous Yogic sun salutations are the perfect way to facilitate this.

Practising several rounds of sun salutations can powerfully awaken the body and induce discernible gains in the levels of energy and vitality we experience. The health benefits of regular sun salutations are profound, helping to remove stiffness and heaviness in the body, optimise circulation and flexibility and stimulate the lymphatic and immune systems while also helping to elevate mood and increase the secretion of our feel-good hormones.

The practice of morning sun salutations in this way should not be viewed as a morning workout. It doesn't require you to break sweat or get out of breath. It is simply a gentle flow through a sequence of energising yoga asanas (poses). However, if you so wish, you can perform these sun salutations for longer or embed them into another yoga flow for a prolonged or more intense morning workout if you know that works for you. For a free five-minute instructional video that breaks down each move of a sun salutation and culminates with the full sequence, see Sun Salutation Sequence in the online resources found at www.mind-body-medical.co.uk/becomingexceptional.

## 5. Breakfast

Once the yoga flow is completed, that marks the end of the morning routine. All that is left to do is eat a healthy and nourishing breakfast that will set you up for the day while also saturating your body with a variety of powerful anti-cancer compounds. Use the nutritional advice explored in chapter 5 to inform this and don't forget to check out the recipes found in the online meal plan for some great tasting anti-cancer breakfast options. (See Recipes and Meal Plan at www.mind-body-medical.co.uk/becomingexceptional.)

And that's it. An effortless flow of transformative practices performed during the unique time of Brahma muhurta, all condensed into the Ayurvedic optimal morning routine. It can take a while to figure out how this routine works best for you and how to tweak and modify it so that it feels natural and easy, but, once you start living this routine each morning, the impacts are as profound as they are discernible. With this covered, we are now ready to focus on the next vital aspect of dinacharya, and that's circadian nutrition.

## Circadian Nutrition: When We Eat Is Just as Important as What We Eat

As we explored in chapter 5, the food we nourish our body with represents one of the most important aspects of cancer survivorship. However, in the Ayurvedic framework, *when* we eat is regarded as being just as important as *what* we eat. This is because in the framework of dinacharya, our ability to optimally digest food peaks and troughs throughout the day. We want to put food into our body when we are best able to digest it and minimise the consumption of food when we are least able to digest it.

Modern-day evidence fully supports this notion, identifying that the human digestive system, including the cells of the liver, gut and pancreas, are all governed by an inbuilt twenty-four-hour circadian clock.[53] If we eat in a way that supports proper circadian alignment in our digestive system, it helps ensure that our digestive mechanisms are able to effectively and efficiently process our food in a way that allows us to fully and completely benefit from the anti-cancer nutritional compounds we are eating. Circadian research suggests that our digestive system is primed to receive most of its food in the early to mid-part of the day, and less food as we move towards evening. Fascinating research now shows how important a role this circadian alignment plays in the context of nutrition.

Consider this. A study conducted at Harvard University gave young adults exactly the same meal at 8 am and then again twelve hours later at 8 pm. Despite the nutritional make-up of the meal being identical, the evening meal induced a much higher and clinically significant increase in blood glucose levels.[54] The meal itself hadn't changed, but the time of eating changed the effects of the meal. On the surface, this looks like a relatively insignificant response in respect of the focus and aims of this book. However, it's not.

Elevated blood glucose induces a concurrent increase in a growth hormone called insulin-like growth factor-1 (IGF-1). The evidence shows that IGF-1 acts as a potent and fast-working growth stimulant for cancer cells.[55] So much so that there is even evidence to suggest that higher IGF-1 levels are a predictor of increased mortality in those with cancer.[56] As such, ensuring balanced blood glucose levels through the day is a key metabolic target for those living with cancer. And in this respect, eating times are of vital importance.

Fortunately, Ayurveda has long advocated a schedule of eating that ensures proper nutritional circadian alignment in this way. Interestingly, it is worth noting that so too did most communities before the Industrial Revolution. For example, in seventeenth-century rural Britain, the biggest meals were consumed at breakfast and lunch, with a much smaller meal consumed early in the evening, around 6 pm. This is a pattern of eating that is still followed by many rural European societies who still adhere to a traditional way of life, particularly in the mountainous regions of France and Italy. And yet for many of us, the reverse is true.

Because of societal changes induced by the Industrial Revolution, the biggest meal of the day has shifted from afternoon lunch to evening dinner, after we have returned from school and work – it is only then that we have time to cook a proper meal and access to a kitchen to do so. The implications of this shift have left most of us in a chronic state of circadian disruption. This is because come the evening, the master clock in our brain is telling us that it will soon be bedtime, and thus begins to shut down the activity of our metabolic and digestive mechanisms because it doesn't anticipate, from a circadian perspective, eating at this time. But the peripheral clocks in our gut and digestive system are having to 'fire up' to deal with a large evening meal.

This misalignment between the commands of the master clock in our brain and the individual clocks in our gut causes a significant state of circadian dysfunction. So much so that eating in this way has now been shown to be a leading risk factor for higher levels of body fat and obesity, increased rates of type 2 diabetes, increased inflammation, poorer immunity, mood dysfunction, fatigue and a whole host of other metabolic ailments, all of which are relevant and important in the context of cancer survivorship. It therefore becomes imperative that we focus not only on the adoption of an evidence-based anti-cancer diet, but also on *when* in the day we are eating the foods that make up this diet. To facilitate this, we can turn to the eating schedule so strongly advocated by Ayurveda, which is as follows.

## Breakfast

Ideally, aim to eat breakfast before 8 am, when the body is metabolically and digestively primed to receive food. Eating breakfast in this way is important as it provides the energy and nourishment the body needs to start the day well and to sustain us until lunchtime. It also allows us to consume a heavy dose of anti-cancer foods early in the day.

## Lunch

Try to eat lunch every day between 12 pm and 1 pm and, where possible, aim to make this the biggest meal of the day. This will help to entrain your circadian rhythm on a daily basis while ensuring you are putting the largest and most nutrient-dense meal into the body when your agni, or digestive capacity, is strongest. By having breakfast and lunch at these times, you ensure that you eat the majority of your calories in the first part of the day, which has consistently been shown to induce better digestive, metabolic and gut health regulation, including better blood glucose balance.

## Dinner

Aim to eat dinner around 6 pm and definitely no later than 7 pm. Eating any later than this can cause significant circadian misalignment. We also want to ensure that our evening meal is nutrient dense but also much lighter because our digestive capacity is significantly weaker around this time, so we want to honour this by eating foods that are much easier to digest.

## Adopt the '12–3' Model

Eating using the schedule described above also ensures that we harness the power of the '12–3' model on a daily basis. This means eating all of our calories in a maximum twelve-hour time frame with the last calorie at least three hours before bed. The impacts of this upon a raft of physiological and metabolic variables relevant to cancer survivorship are significant because it ensures a minimum twelve-hour fasting period in every twenty-four-hour cycle while also helping to prevent any circadian disruption.

## Consistency is Key

Aim to eat your meals at the same time every day. To effectively process food, your body has to release a whole cascade of digestive hormones, secretions and enzymes prior to eating. If we constantly change the time we eat, it becomes impossible for our body clock to predict when we will next be eating and the whole system moves out of sync. Eating at the same time every day allows our circadian clock to accurately predict when it will next receive food and thus be best placed to receive and digest it. A brilliant marker of moving into nutritional circadian alignment in this way is that we experience a subtle sense of physical hunger before each meal.

### A Word on Weight Loss

If you have lost weight that you need to regain, you can modify the above schedule slightly to allow for the addition of an extra meal. I have used this approach regularly and have found it to be very effective at facilitating healthy weight gain. To do so, try eating breakfast at 8 am, an early lunch around 11 am, a second lunch around 3 pm and then dinner around 6 pm to 7 pm.

## Sacred Sleep: Ayurveda's Optimal Evening Routine for Blissful Sleep

In our discussions around the importance of dinacharya thus far, we have focused exclusively on harnessing the power of the solar cycle of the day and living in a way that aligns the microcosm of our body with the macrocosm of the wider world. But like the yin and yang of traditional Chinese medicine, the entire universe is made up of opposites; hot and cold, wet and dry, light and dark, old and young, healthy and unhealthy and an infinite array of other pairings. And so too with the circadian rhythm, both in our bodies and in the wider world. To fully thrive during the solar cycle of the day, we must support and prioritise an equal thriving during the lunar cycle of the night. And to do that we must consciously prioritise sleep as much as any other self-care practice we adopt. To emphasise just how importantly Ayurveda views the concept of deep, restorative sleep, consider this beautiful verse from the *Charaka Samhita*, one of the most sacred texts within the Ayurvedic framework:

> Our quota of happiness and unhappiness, nourishment and emaciation, strength and debility, sexual power and impotence, knowledge and ignorance and, in fact, life and death, are all dependent on sleep itself.

The modern-day published clinical evidence very much supports the vehemence with which Ayurveda prioritises the importance of sleep in the pursuit of radical health. It has long been known that chronically disrupted sleep patterns are an independent risk factor for a whole raft of diseases, including heart disease, diabetes, obesity, Alzheimer's and much else besides.[57] Similarly, chronically impaired sleep can negatively impact upon a whole host of physiological and psychological variables relevant to cancer survivorship. For example, sleep dysfunction can significantly alter the workings of our metabolic, hormonal and immune systems in a damaging way, resulting in chronically impaired immune function and the promotion of systemic long-term inflammation,[58] both of which are directly implicated in poorer cancer survivorship outcomes.[59] Similarly, poor sleep patterns can decrease the circulating levels of melatonin in our body. This is crucial because melatonin has been shown to play an important role in the suppression of several of the primary hallmarks of cancer promotion.[60] Last but not least, experiencing poor sleep can greatly reduce the quality of life in those living with cancer. Specifically, it has been shown to induce much lower levels of energy and vitality, poorer mood states and higher levels of anxiety and depression.[61] This relationship is so important that the National Comprehensive Cancer Network in the US updated their guidelines to ensure that clinicians proactively screen those with cancer for potential sleep disorders as an integral part of their survivorship protocols.[62] Put simply, cultivating optimal sleeping patterns is a prerequisite for experiencing increased health and vitality in the body, both generically and in the specific context of cancer survivorship. And Ayurveda gifts us with some beautifully holistic advice for doing so.

## 1. Be Consistent with Your Waking and Sleeping Times

Waking at the correct time of the morning acts as the lynchpin for blissful sleep. This is because early morning exposure to sunlight sets an internal stop-watch in the brain, instructing it to start producing melatonin – the hormone most responsible for sleep regulation – around fourteen hours later.[63] So, if for example, we awaken bright and early at 6am and immediately open the blinds and expose our retina to early morning light, the hormonal upshot of this is that around fourteen hours later, at around 8 pm, melatonin production will kick in perfectly. This then supports a deep and restful sleep that night, with one caveat; we must aim to be in bed and asleep before 10 pm. By this time, melatonin will be working its magic and we should be feeling naturally sleepy. By keeping a consistent bedtime in this way, the body can predict when sleep is expected and can optimally regulate itself to support this. Thus, the most important practice we can adopt to enjoy the transformative benefits of deep, blissful sleep is to maintain a consistent and circadian-aligned wake/sleep cycle. The impacts of doing so truly can be profound.

## 2. Promote Kapha in the Evening

From 6 pm to 10 pm in the evening kapha dosha naturally starts building in the body. Because this build-up is responsible for the promotion of deep sleep, we want to further aid the promotion of kapha via our practices and routines. A great way to do this is to massage a warm, heavy oil such as sesame oil (which is inherently kapha building) onto the soles of the feet, shoulders, neck and earlobes. Spending a few minutes mindfully performing this ritual before bed is incredibly calming and relaxing and can really help support more restful sleep.

## 3. Avoid Stimulation

As the day comes to a close and night falls it is important that we minimise our exposure to any form of stimulation. Stimulatory activities such as exercise, eating, working, scrolling through social media, checking emails, watching distressing news on the television and drinking caffeine or alcohol all force the cells of our body to 'fire up' when the master clock in the brain is telling them to 'wind down' in preparation for the coming night. This misalignment causes the body to secrete cortisol into the blood so that we are better prepared to deal with whatever it is that has stimulated us. This release of cortisol into the blood will leave us feeling wide awake and often a little wired. The unnatural secretion of nighttime cortisol also powerfully suppresses the activity of melatonin. This creates a 'double whammy', which ultimately makes it incredibly difficult, if not impossible, to enjoy optimal sleep that night. Thus, as much as possible, ensure all activities past 8 pm are ones that have a calming and relaxing effect on your body and mind, such as a relaxing bath, reading, listening to music, meditation or the practice of a specific type of sleep-promoting yoga called yoga nidra, rather than excitatory ones. Yoga nidra is the simplest and easiest of all the different types of yoga practice and one that doesn't involve yoga sequences or holding poses. Instead, yoga nidra is practised lying down, and induces a profound sense of calm in both the body and mind that paves the way for a deep and restful night's sleep.

## 4. Set a Screen Curfew

This is vital. The darkness that falls as we move into the evening is the signal for the SCN in the brain to instruct the body that the day has ended and nighttime operations needs to commence. However, exposing our eyes to intense blue light in the form of smart phones, tablets and computers in the evening causes immense circadian dysfunction because the SCN in the brain is communicating to the body that it is nighttime while at the same time our individual cellular clocks are reporting back that it's daytime due to them being exposed to artificial blue light. Countless studies now show that the circadian misalignment caused by nighttime blue light significantly disrupts melatonin production and causes poorer sleep profiles.[64] To circumvent this problem, it is a good idea to set an 8 pm curfew on all blue light. If you must use devices after this time, use blue light-suppressing glasses, which, to some extent, reduce the risks.

## 5: Optimise Your Sleeping Environment

The environment in our bedroom has a significant impact upon our mental state in relation to preparing our body for optimal sleep. Ensure that your bedroom is calming, inviting and peaceful and try to remove anything that creates a stimulatory energy such as TVs, laptops or phones. Similarly, untidiness, clutter and mess all invoke the stimulating energies of vata. This can leave us feeling unsettled, anxious and ungrounded, which are not the qualities we desire to support optimal sleep. Thus, ensure your room is tidy and calming and ideally decorated in colours and themes that you personally find grounding and relaxing.

## 6. Meditation

In the Ayurvedic optimal morning routine discussed earlier, we explored the importance of starting the day with meditation. The same is also true of the evening. If you find it hard to switch off and fall asleep, this is often because the mind is too active. Meditation is the perfect antidote to this and clinical research now advocates the use of evening meditation as a proven remedy for sleep dysfunction.[65] Thus embedding a fifteen- to twenty-minute meditation sitting on your bed before turning the lights off can really help ground the mind and prepare you for deep, restful sleep.

## 7. Set a 9 pm 'Withdrawal'

Last but by no means least, aim to set a 9 pm withdrawal. By this time of the evening, the master clock in our brain will be instructing the body that the day has ended. The time for productivity, stress, work, physical activity, eating, stimulation and virtually everything else is over. We need to honour this. The 9 pm withdrawal is a great way of doing so as it allows us to consciously and proactively withdraw from the outer world and all its demands. At this time of the evening, there should be nothing left for us to do. Our sole focus should be on using this last hour of the day to prepare for, and consciously cultivate, blissful sleep, and so the 9 pm withdrawal is a practice I would strongly encourage you to adopt. It can allow you to build a powerful evening routine, which could involve going into the beautiful, peaceful sanctuary of your bedroom at 9 pm, dimming the lights or perhaps lighting a candle and performing the kapha-inducing oil massage in a mindful way (see Promote Kapha in the Evening on page 162) with some calming music playing in the background. Great options here include nature sounds, such as falling rain, wind chimes or whale song. Once finished, move on to a grounding twenty-minute meditation, perhaps with the same music playing, to leave you feeling heavy, tired and deeply relaxed. Then perhaps say a quick prayer of gratitude for the day that has just passed, mentally affirm the brilliance of tomorrow, switch off the lights, and enjoy a blissful sleep after a day lived fully in the magic of full and complete circadian alignment.

##  Chapter Affirmations for My Journey to Becoming Exceptional

1. I consciously see myself as an integral part of the natural world all around me and acknowledge my need to align with nature's inbuilt circadian rhythms.
2. I commit to unleashing the power of rta and circadian alignment in the physiology of my body by harnessing the power of Brahma muhurta.
3. I recognise the importance of the Ayurvedic Optimal Morning Routine and commit to individualising this routine and then complying with it as an integral aspect of my overarching survivorship protocol.
4. I commit to harnessing the often-untapped benefits of chrono-nutrition and nourishing my body with potent anti-cancer foods at the times of the day it can best benefit from them.
5. I acknowledge the importance of blissful sleep and commit to structuring my evening routine to allow for this.
6. **Summary Affirmation:** Each and every day I unleash the transformative powers of circadian medicine as I powerfully and purposefully progress along the path of becoming exceptional.

# CHAPTER NINE

# Awakening the Body's Inner Pharmacy

## *The Sensory Pathways of Healing*

*We have a pharmacy inside of us that is absolutely exquisite. It is able to make the right medicine, for the precise time, for the right target organ – with no side effects.*

DEEPAK CHOPRA, *The Healing Self*

Before we begin our journey into exploring the concept of awakening the body's inner pharmacy, which for me represents one of the most holistic frameworks of healing gifted to us by Ayurveda, I would firstly like you to put this book down for a few minutes and contemplate the following:

How has your day been today up to this very minute in time? What things have brought you joy, happiness or a sense of meaning? Have you seen or spoken to the people you love the most this morning? How did kissing your partner or cuddling a loved one make you feel? If you have been out today for a walk or run, how did the environment affect you or make you feel? Were you walking in a beautiful forest, an unending sandy beach or the natural oasis of an inner-city park? Did you get to watch the sunrise and, if so, what impact did it have upon you? Perhaps you have listened to music and felt your mood or energy increase through doing so. Or perhaps earlier today you mindfully brewed a beautiful fresh pot of coffee or an aromatic herbal tea and enjoyed the aromas and anticipation of sitting down somewhere quietly to savour it. Ultimately, has this day, up to this very minute, been good or bad, joyful or frustrating, happy or sad, positive or challenging?

Really connect with the deepest sensations and emotions in your body and mind right now and tune in to what 'things' have actually made you feel this way? For example, if kissing your child first thing this morning made you feel a deep sense of love and gratitude, how did doing so actually and tangibly create these emotions? Or if you consciously woke earlier to watch a striking sunrise that left you feeling awestruck and alive, how did doing so actually induce these tangible alterations in the emotional workings of your mind? Extend this thought process further and think about the exact mechanisms by which any external 'thing' outside of your body is able to directly, powerfully and often very quickly alter the ways in which you think, behave and feel in your body and mind. The only way any external thing – be that a beautiful view, the presence of a loved one, an uplifting book or a moving poem – can facilitate these kinds of changes is via the unique actions of our five senses. These senses – our ability to see, hear, smell, touch and taste – are the *only* ways in which we can directly interact and engage with the outer world. We can think of them as an immensely powerful portal for facilitating the dynamic exchange of information from the outer world of the environment directly into the inner world of our body. And the content and make-up of this information will *always* impact upon how our body and mind function at the physiological, biochemical and emotional level.

Imagine it's a beautifully warm summer's afternoon and you are out walking in your village or town. Passing by one particular house, you smell the uniquely sweet scent of freshly mown grass. As you breathe in this immensely evocative smell, an almost instantaneous flood of memories springs forth of joyful and innocent summer days when you were a child. Often, these kinds of memories can evoke an almost palpable bubbling up of positive emotional states, such as happiness, security and love. And when we smell that scent and experience those memories, the emotions that stem from them don't simply remain in our mind. They go on to stimulate a cascade of quantifiable healing responses in the physiology of the body. Specifically, they can go on to increase the secretion of our healing feel-good hormones, lower our harmful stress hormones, reduce inflammation, optimise immune activity and lower blood pressure, to name but a few. In other words, the connection between an outside event (the smell of freshly cut grass) enters the body via the portal of the senses (the olfactory nerves in the nose) and then induces a specific emotional response, which then in turn goes on to activate a variety of physiological mechanisms relevant to healing and improved physical and emotional wellbeing.

Viewed in this light, we can see that our five senses, or more accurately the stimuli that they are exposed to, afford us access to an immensely powerful therapeutic modality that we can consciously press into service in our quest to control and optimise the workings of our body in the direction of healing. And within the Ayurvedic tradition, this healing potential lying dormant within the five senses is revered with such intensity that it has been developed into a therapeutic framework in and of itself called *tanmatra chikitsa*.

Tanmatra chikitsa is based upon the belief that all of the tens of thousands of sensory impressions we experience every day play a profound role in the way in which our body works and functions and whether this functionality is healing or harming. So, just as the food we eat goes on to create the physical reality of our bodily tissues, so too do the sounds we hear, the sights we observe, the scents we smell and the physical touch we experience. According to the science of tanmatra chikitsa, if we want to stimulate healing and experience greater physical and emotional wellbeing, we can proactively and consciously control the sensory impressions we expose ourselves to in such a way as to cultivate these specific objectives. For example, imagine you knew that listening to the sound of gently falling rain was incredibly relaxing and calming for you. Knowing this, you could choose to play such sounds quietly in the background when you are working, cooking or doing housework. What would be the benefit of this? The benefit would be that your auditory nerves would pick up on these sounds that are so deeply relaxing to you and through so doing activate the parasympathetic nervous system, which is responsible for the activation of specific healing responses in your body. Thus, with no active effort on your part, you would be powerfully altering your physiology in a way that supports better immune, hormone and nervous system status simply by pressing into service the healing potential found in our sense of sound. And this is not a small gain; published clinical research now shows that listening to nature sounds (among others) can powerfully increase the number of immune cells in the body and the intelligence with which they work,[1] which, as we have previously explored, is of fundamental importance in the context of cancer survivorship.

Furthermore, the power of sensory-driven healing is that it is working *all* of the time. We may typically only meditate once or twice a day, eat two or three times a day or exercise once a day. But our senses are being exposed to an infinite array of stimuli every second of our lives in waking state (and in sleep too). If we can consciously control and filter these sensory stimuli, we can use the framework of tanmatra chikitsa to unleash powerful and proven healing responses in the body.

As a relatively extreme but illuminating hypothetical example of the significance of this, try imagining the transformative impacts you would experience in your mind and body if you were to spend one whole day (or longer) living in an environment filled almost exclusively with sensory stimuli that you associate with bliss and happiness. For me personally, this would look like a simple but comfortable log cabin somewhere in the European Alps in the summer. Surrounded by alpine meadows bejewelled with wildflowers, there would be a beautiful river flowing close by, towering peaks in the distance and the complete absence of any sign of humanity. My days would be spent walking and hiking in this paradise of natural beauty with those I love the most. Unhurried days spent reading, cooking nourishing food, listening to the beautiful symphony of the rushing river, wild birds and the warm wind swaying the pine forests. There would be amazing conversations interspersed with prolonged periods of silence. There would be fresh air, the complete absence of digital distractions, sun-kissed skin and a glowing sense of tiredness each evening that paved the way for deep, blissful and rejuvenating sleep.

In this sensory utopia, it is almost impossible to quantify the healing impacts that would be unleashed within the body. And this unleashing would be facilitated, almost exclusively, through and by the sensory stimuli we are consciously exposing ourselves to. Virtually every minute of every day, these sights, smells, sounds, tastes and kinaesthetic experiences would saturate the workings of every cell of our body with molecules of happiness, gratitude, wonder and the sheer exuberance of being alive. In this molecular soup of positivity, the only option open to the body is one of healing. It is for this reason that retreating into nature in the quest for healing informs a core practice in virtually every single system of traditional medicine in the world. And while booking a sensory retreat such as this is a very realistic goal for lots of people (and one that I personally prioritise heavily), we also need to learn how to harness the impacts of sensory healing in our normal day-to-day lives via the subtle and conscious modification of what we expose our senses to.

As a clinical modality, this is the entire goal and aim of tanmatra chikitsa. And it is through the doors of tanmatra chikitsa that we are able to proactively enter into and awaken the inner pharmacy that is an inherent part of the human body and activate it in the direction of healing. Because for more than five thousand years, Ayurveda has stressed that within each and every one of us, often lying dormant and untapped, is an extensive array of potent and naturally occurring hormones, immunemodulators, neuropeptides and chemicals that the body can unleash to radically enhance our health, wellbeing and healing potential. This concept of awakening the body's inner pharmacy is one that is now unequivocally acknowledged in Western academic medicine, which shows that the body can create natural equivalents to most types of pharmaceutical drugs such as pain killers, antihypertensives, anti-inflammatories and much else besides. The aim of this chapter is to provide guidance and instruction on how we can use the portal of our senses of smell, sight and sound as a vehicle for powerful inner healing. The reason for omitting the other two senses – taste and touch – is that by following the nutritional advice found in chapter 5 and the self-massage practice advocated in chapter 8, you will be already be harnessing the benefits of these two senses in a clinically active way.

## Healing Sounds

Sound waves are able to impact the workings of our mind, body and cells in powerful ways. As an extreme example of this, imagine the response in your body if a deafening crash were to go off behind you unexpectedly. It would most likely make you physically jump into the air, increase your heart rate and possibly even induce a sweat response on the palms of your hands, forehead or back. All of these acute, observable changes in the body and mind have been induced by nothing more than invisible waves of sound. From this example we can clearly see that sound can almost instantly impact upon our physiology. Our focus needs to be on learning how to harness this potential for physiological regulation specifically in the context of healing.

This is a mechanism that we as a species have been consciously harnessing since time immemorial; anthropological research shows that our species' earliest designated healers, the shamans of East Africa, almost certainly used rhythmic drum beats to invoke healing as part of their elaborate medicinal rituals.[2] And so, too, in Ayurveda, which attributes to the power of sound not just the potential to heal but also the existence of the entire universe. This is because in the Vedas (the ancient texts in which the original principles of

Ayurveda were recorded) the initial vibration that brought everything into existence was the sound 'om'. This is why om is called the 'cosmic sound' and why one of the sound healing techniques explored later in this chapter uses this sacred sound as a specific form of healing intervention.

Fast-forward to the twenty-first century and robust and compelling clinical evidence supports the use of sound as a therapeutic tool to help mobilise the healing mechanisms of the body. It is now known that sound therapy can significantly alter the activity of brainwaves in a way that supports improved emotional and psychological health, including higher states of peace, calm and emotional security.[3] These neurological and emotional alterations are in turn able to directly modify the functionality of a whole raft of important physiological health parameters, including improved immune function and immune counts, a reduction in stress hormones, an increased secretion of dopamine and serotonin and lower inflammatory states.[4]

The clinical interest around the potential application of sound as a supportive therapy in cancer survivorship has gained real traction over the last decade. And the results of this research are highly promising. For example, it has been observed that sound therapy can reduce psychological distress and fear, boost mood and positivity, lower chemotherapy-induced anxiety, improve overall levels of functional quality of life and even reduce the severity and prevalence of pain in those with cancer.[5] In light of these clear and immutable benefits, the integration of sound therapy into your survivorship protocol is highly recommended. Here are some fantastic ways of doing so.

## Nature Sounds

Perhaps more than any other form of sound, the music that the natural world gifts to us so abundantly and so freely is arguably the most therapeutically powerful of all sound therapy. This is because unlike the music we create that has been produced from the minds of humans, in the Eastern tradition the primordial sounds of nature spring forth from the very mind of God. Because of this, they are said to possess unique healing properties.

I am sure that most of us can intuitively associate with this whenever we enter into direct communion with nature. Whether sitting peacefully in our garden listening to the singing birds, walking through a beautiful wood and connecting with the sound of the wind as it rustles the trees, losing ourselves in the almost hypnotic rhythms of gently breaking waves on the beach or when lying in bed and listening to the pitter-patter of rain on the roof, these are all deeply calming sounds. In my experience, these types of sounds are the ones that resonate most powerfully with us and thus are the ones that possess the most dormant healing potential. They are also a joy to engage with as doing so requires us to retract from our overly digitalised and busy lives and enter into and connect with the slower rhythms of nature.

To harness these benefits, try to schedule regular retreats into nature with the sole intent of accessing its healing power. Visit woods and forests and simply sit somewhere peaceful, close your eyes and lose yourself in the sounds to be found there – falling leaves, the wind, the summer hum of crickets, the birdsong and so much more. Or visit a powerfully flowing river and become absorbed in its song as it courses over rapids or waterfalls. You could make a trip to the beach and enjoy the sun on your face, the heady aroma of salty air, and immerse yourself in the hypnotic infinitude of the breaking waves.

Connecting with experiences such as these on a regular basis, through all of the seasons, can have a powerfully transformative impact upon our emotional outlook, mood, energy, optimism and general quality of life. Additionally, you can also find a huge variety of nature sounds to download or purchase online, which will allow you to harness their benefits at home or when you are unable to physically get out into the natural world. Later in the chapter, we will also explore the concept of forest bathing, which is a fantastic practice for tapping into all of these benefits in a more structured way.

## Chanting

Virtually every spiritual and religious tradition in the world has called upon the transformative power of chanting as a tool to induce deeper spiritual experiences and to elevate the life energy of those using such practices. And for good reason; the deep resonations and melodious repetitions inherent in chanting can have an almost hypnotic effect on us. There has been much clinical research around the benefits of chanting as a specific sub-set of sound therapy and this research shows that chants are able to induce very unique changes in our brainwaves, heart-coherence and mood.[6] These all combine to help activate the healing and rejuvenating activity of our healing parasympathetic nervous system.

Harnessing these benefits is as simple as finding the type of chant that most deeply resonates with you and listening to this on a regular basis. Personally,

I find Gregorian chants, which originate from the Christian tradition, to be immensely powerful to the point that they are able to make us temporarily forget ourselves and all sense of time and space. Similarly, from the Vedic tradition come forth equally famous chants such as the Gayatri, which is a beautiful sung mantra that is deeply moving. All of these chants are easy to source online and are freely available on YouTube. We can also create our own chants. Earlier, we mentioned the 'om' vibration as being the most important chant or sound in the Vedic tradition. We can use this during our meditation practice, or simply as a chanting exercise, by slowly and deeply humming the om sound. Doing so requires us to take a slow, deep and controlled in-breath and then on the out-breath hum the sound om (pronounced 'ommm'). When doing this, you should feel a deep vibration all along the back of the mouth and throat. This is a beautiful practice to try and one that builds a bridge between the impacts and benefits of sound therapy and meditation.

## *Music*

In addition to the use of nature sounds and chanting, we can also use general music in a therapeutic way. And the power of this approach is that we can use different types of music to elicit different physiological and emotional responses. For example, if you are feeling tired and sluggish in the morning, you could consciously listen to more energising and stimulating music to help fire up your energy. Or, if you are feeling very anxious or stressed, you could proactively choose to listen to music that you find very calming and grounding. It is good practice to begin to explore, and perhaps to jot down or create a playlist of, the different types of music you enjoy that affect you in different ways. Then, whenever you are experiencing an undesirable state – be that fatigue, stress, fear or anger – you would have a selection of pre-prepared music that would help alleviate such states.

Similarly, you can find and build playlists to help you cope emotionally with difficult clinical events. For example, if you find that MRIs, CT scans or the chemotherapy treatment centre awaken strong negative emotional responses (which they so often do) you can use music to offset and antidote this. Even better, you could consciously choose to play specific music every time you meditate, practise yoga or perform a self-massage. Through this, your subconscious mind will associate that specific music with a deep sense of relaxation and calm. If you were then to play the same music in the MRI tunnel, or in the waiting room prior to scan results, it would trigger the same relaxation in your body via a Pavlovian response. This can really help to dial down the severity of acute stress in these types of challenging clinical settings.

## Healing Images

Our power of sight is often referred to as our 'sovereign sense' because it is the one that we as a species living in the twenty-first century typically value, use and rely on the most. And because of this, the things we visually connect with over the course of each day play a leading role in regulating the physiological and biochemical workings of the body. For example, imagine it's the weekend and you are all alone in your home watching a crime thriller on the television. The film is approaching its scariest part, the tension is building and you find yourself almost unable to watch. Your logical self 'knows' it's only a film, but that doesn't stop your brain reacting to the anticipated fear as if it were real. If, in this situation, you were to be tested in the laboratory, you would find a real-time increase in the stress hormone cortisol, an increase in heart rate and blood pressure and the activation of the fight or flight response in the biochemistry of the body. These would be observable and measurable changes brought about by nothing more than a series of images on a TV screen.

Contrast this experience with one at the other end of the therapeutic spectrum. Imagine it's a warm summer's evening and you are sitting outside, perhaps next to a crackling firepit, as the sun sets. As darkness approaches, a massive full moon rises above the horizon, leaving you spellbound. And as the darkness continues to fall, and the fire slowly burns down, an infinity of stars reveal themselves in the night sky. The peace, energy and beauty of the moment is beguiling and leaves you feeling safe, reassured and awestruck. The impacts of such an experience would profoundly alter the workings of the body at the physiological and biochemical level; immunity would increase, stress hormones would drop and we would be flooded with mood-elevating feel-good hormones.

The gulf between the body's response to these two different experiences, and the harming or healing impacts they produce, is simply the net result of the visual stimuli observed. And herein lies the key to harnessing the healing power of sight; as much as possible, only allow into your world, and the environments you occupy, sights and images that nourish you and make you feel happy, healthy, safe and alive. Here are some great practices for doing so:

- Saturate your home with photographs of those you love and past memories that fill you with a sense of gratitude, happiness and health.
- Make every facet of your home a sensory delight in terms of decorations, colours, ornaments and furnishings; ensure that every room you frequent elevates your energy via the visual stimuli contained there.
- Regularly gaze at images that evoke an excitement for the future – holidays to book, places to visit, people to see and memories to make. You could make a vision board of these images and gaze upon them regularly as a way of building positive excitement and expectation around the future. (By the way, this is a practice that further supports the goal-setting imagery techniques explored in chapter 4 – see Practising Goal-Setting Imagery on page 58.)
- Hang beautiful works of art upon your walls that fill you with delight and inspire you to gaze upon them.
- Explore lots of different environments – beaches, forests, mountains, rivers – and saturate your sense of sight with the abundant splendour found there.
- Delight in the beauty of the natural world all around you; the flowers in your garden, the birds on your fence, your faithful dog curled up on his bed.
- Shower your home with vases of flowers that evoke a sense of splendour.
- Few sights are as mesmerising as natural flames, so try lighting a firepit and spend an evening every so often gazing into this, perhaps joined by your family for an evening of digital-free companionship and contemplation.
- Actively seek out captivating sights, such as sunrises and sunsets, full moons, star-filled nights, waterfalls and snowcapped peaks.
- Make time to visit places that contain sights that you love; sport matches, art galleries, zoos, the playground with your children or grandchildren and myriad other places.
- If you have a religious practice, gaze at devotional art or images, such as a crucifix or statue, and connect deeply with this.

In short, try to ensure that your days, as much as possible, are spent in the presence of sights that evoke a tangible sense of awe, beauty and wonder. If you can do that, every day will be an effortless harnessing of the healing powers of sight.

## A Word on Geometric Visual Healing

In the Vedic and Yogic traditions, certain geometric designs and images have long been used as a means of unleashing the healing energy of sight. There are many options available to facilitate this, but a particularly beautiful one, which is a joy to create when done mindfully, and even more joyful to gaze upon, is as follows:

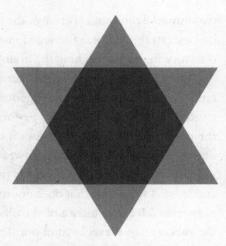

Figure 9.1. The shatkona yantra hexagram.

1. Get a beautiful wooden tray and onto this pour some plain flour.
2. Then, with your finger, draw an image like the one in figure 9.1 into the flour.
3. Place a small bowl of water in this middle of this image.
4. In this bowl of water, float a small tealight and light this.
5. If possible, also add a small flower or petal.
6. Place this somewhere prominent and gaze at it frequently.

This type of creation is said to possess immense healing energy because it contains all five of the great elements: ether and air (which is all around us), fire (via the candle), water (in the bowl) and earth (as represented by the solidity of the bowl or the flower, if used). In doing so, it is said to naturally harmonise and balance all three doshas and thus the entire workings of the body. Aside from this, it is also a beautifully aesthetic design that is a pleasure to stop and gaze upon every so often.

## Healing Aromas

Evolutionarily speaking, smell is the oldest and most primitive of the five senses and one that, until relatively recently, was our most dominant sense. For millions of years, our pre-human ancestors were neurologically hardwired to rely heavily on their incredibly acute sense of smell to survive and prosper. Indeed, until *Homo sapiens* emerged as a new species around two hundred thousand years ago, the majority of the grey matter making up our ancestral brain was funnelled into the direct and specific processing of olfactory messages reaching the brain from the nose.

This is best illustrated by the fact that the olfactory neuroreceptor gene family is the largest in our entire genome.[7] In this way, our sense of smell was trusted to help us successfully perform all the activities that were vital for the preservation of life: the location of food and water, avoiding predators, finding a sexual mate, predicting weather, organising social hierarchies and much else besides. Today, sight has overtaken smell as our most important and trusted sense, but that does not mean we have shaken off the evolutionarily embedded dominance of the olfactory system. While often working at the subconscious level beyond our direct awareness, our sense of smell still exerts massive influence over our mind, emotions, physiology and healing responses. This is because when we smell a pleasing or evocative scent, the odour molecules making up that scent are breathed in via the nostrils, where they then attach to the olfactory sensory neuroreceptors located behind the bridge of the nose. From here, the scent molecules are transformed into nerve impulses that are delivered, via nerve fibres, directly into the olfactory bulb. This is crucial because the olfactory bulb directly connects to key areas of the brain, most importantly the limbic system.

Consisting of the most ancient parts of the brain, such as the hippocampus, hypothalamus and amygdala, the limbic system exerts immense influence upon the regulation of both our physiology and our emotions. For example, the limbic system is responsible for the regulation of blood pressure, breathing rates, heart rate, hormone regulation, digestion, immune function and status, and mood. And because the limbic system is so evolutionarily suggestible to the impact of scents, we can proactively use smells to consciously modulate the workings of the limbic system in the direction of healing. And to do that, we simply need to know how to use smells in a specific way. For the sake of clarity and simplicity, there are two general ways of doing so: 1) essential oils; and 2) natural smells. Each of these are explored in turn below.

## Using Essential Oils in the Quest for Healing

Herbal essential oils provide us with an incredibly powerful, easy-to-use and evidence-based vehicle for harnessing the healing power of smell. This is a modality of healing that humans have utilised for millennia, with the first systematically documented accounts being found in ancient Egypt around 2800 BCE.[8] Around eight hundred years later, the first Ayurvedic treatise on the use of essential oils emerged in the famous text, the *Charika Samhita*. In this, one can find detailed instructions for the distillation and condensation of the volatile essential oils found in myriad plants and herbs.[9] So important did the application of aromatic medicine become within the Ayurvedic tradition that early Indian medicine men and women were known as *perfumeros* due to the heavy emphasis they placed on aromatic medicine.[10]

To this day, the clinical use of essential oils remains an integral aspect of Ayurvedic medicine and one that has quickly found its way into the arena of Western evidence-based integrative cancer care. Within the National Health Service in the UK, aromatherapy is a recognised and valued form of complementary medicine that is widely offered to those with cancer. And for good reason. There is now compelling evidence to show how the use of essential oils affords clinical efficacy in the management of a whole raft of symptoms commonly experienced by those living with cancer. This includes reducing anxiety,[11] improving sleep duration and quality,[12] alleviating chemotherapy-induced side effects,[13] improving mood and aiding relaxation[14] and reducing the side effects of radiotherapy.[15] Furthermore, there is a growing foundation of exciting research to highlight the cytotoxic (cancer-destroying) potential of essential oils. For instance, essential oils such as eucalyptus, chamomile, verbena, boswellia and thyme have all been shown to induce apoptosis (cancer cell death), slow the proliferation of cancer cell growth, inhibit angiogenesis and suppress tissue invasion rates in many different types of cancer.[16] And while it should be emphasised that this research has been conducted in Petri dishes and mice rather than in humans, it nevertheless suggests real promise in the use of aromatic medicine as part of a robust and all-encompassing integrative cancer survivorship framework.

## How to Use Essential Oils

The best framework I know of for harnessing the healing potential of aromatic medicine in a truly individualised manner is via the wisdom of the doshas. You will remember from our earlier discussions that Ayurveda recognises three mind-body types, called doshas. These are called vata, pitta and kapha. To gain an understanding of your current doshic balance, complete the Vikruti Assessment Questionnaire in appendix 1, on page 219. With this knowledge, you will be best placed to know which specific essential oils you should be using to support your health and wellbeing. For example:

**Vata Dominance:** If you are vata dominant right now, you may be experiencing common vata ailments, such as stress, anxiety, poor sleep, fatigue, constipation, gas, dry skin, weakness or weight loss. Ideal essential oils to use in these instances are grounding and warming options, which include ginger, rose, sandalwood, vanilla, basil and orange.

**Pitta Dominance:** If you are presently pitta dominant, common symptoms such as irritability, anger, short-temperedness, inflammatory digestive and skin diseases, hot flushes or diarrhoea may be dominant. Great essential oil options here include cooling lavender, jasmine, mint, chamomile or ylang-ylang.

**Kapha Dominance:** Lastly, if you sense you are kapha dominant now, you could be experiencing symptoms such as lethargy, tiredness, sluggishness, weight gain, water retention, swelling or congestion. The best essential oil options to help manage these symptoms would include more stimulating eucalyptus, ginger, cloves, juniper and camphor.

If you are experiencing symptoms from two doshas at the same time, you can combine oils that specifically support these two doshas into one oil blend by simply mixing your chosen oils together.

The simplest and easiest way to then use these oils is via an essential oil diffuser. This heats and disperses essential oils into the room via steam. These are incredibly effective as they provide a constant and steady supply of essential oil molecules into the air all around you. Thus if you have the diffuser working when you are reading, watching television, working or anything else, you will be consciously and powerfully harnessing the benefits of aromatic medicine via the simple act of breathing. Therefore, why not try investing in a diffuser and a selection of essential oils based upon your unique preferences and use these regularly as a simple tool for health promotion. A list of recommended suppliers for top-quality essential oils can be found in Essential Oils and Sundries on page 228 in appendix 3.

## Other Healing Scents

While essential oils are without doubt the easiest and most evidence-based means of accessing the healing power of our olfactory system, they are by no means the only way. My preference is to use essential oils regularly but to also ensure we support these with more natural and spontaneous healing aromas.

Remember, the olfactory pathway directly, and virtually instantaneously, regulates the emotional centres of the brain. Any aroma that we find positively evocative, beautiful, pleasant or meaningful will powerfully activate the workings of the brain in the direction of healing – we want to actively facilitate and seek out such aromas. And like shooting stars in the night sky, which are so mesmerising because of their brevity, we need to consciously and proactively seize these types of evocative aromas when they occur.

I will never forget the way this was described to me by a lady with breast cancer, Marion, who was a member of one of the cancer survivorship groups I ran many years ago. Marion was positively euphoric about the impacts that sensory healing was having upon her levels of health and wellbeing, and she gifted us with a great example of how she consciously integrated this into her life. More specifically, she said that of all the smells in the world, her absolute favourite was the smell of fresh rain on dry ground (which, out of interest, is called petrichor). Whenever new rain arrived, rather than cursing the weather, she chose to embrace it as an opportunity for self-elevation by going outside and savouring this most unique of smells. She spoke of her almost childlike joy towards the sensations of rain drops on her bare skin and how she would close her eyes and deeply inhale that wonderful smell. She spoke of how she would become completely absorbed in this experience and through doing so would become more fully alive, mindfully present and powerfully optimistic.

This, to me, is what deep healing looks like as these types of almost transcendental experiences invoke healing responses that are almost impossible to quantify for the simple fact that they exist outside of the limited parameters of science. For this very reason we need to seek them out and utilise them as often as we possibly can. Other similar examples include the beautiful, salty smell of the sea, the heady aroma found uniquely in pine forests (more on this later), freshly cut grass or the unmistakable aroma of summer flowers in full bloom. Seek these out and use them to access the unique healing potential only they can unleash. More controllable examples include the smell of freshly brewed coffee, warm bread straight out of the oven, the freshly washed hair of your child, your partner's perfume or a bouquet of flowers placed on the kitchen table. To stop to consciously engage with these types of smells is to access and unleash the unique benefits of aromatic medicine, which are always there but often missed.

## Forest Bathing: The Ultimate Cancer-Specific Sensory Experience

Before we conclude this chapter, it is crucial to spend a little time exploring the unique sensory healing opportunity gifted to us by the Japanese practice of forest bathing, or *Shinrin-yoku*. And while this practice may have originated in Japan, it powerfully complies with the Ayurvedic concept of tanmatra chikitsa. It provides us with what is arguably the most powerful, immersive and evidence-based practice for harnessing *all* of the different types of sensory healing mechanisms thus far explored in this chapter into one immensely transformative – and in some cases euphoric – practice. Personally speaking, I have taught immersive forest bathing sessions for many years in the South Downs National Park, which lies just north of where I live.

During these sessions, I have seen first-hand just how profound an impact it can have upon the physical and mental wellbeing of those taking part; testimonies include reference to improved sleep, reduced anxiety, increased energy, lower levels of pain, reduced fatigue, and increased positivity and mood. In fact, if I combine these types of first-hand experiences with the published clinical evidence that supports why forest bathing is mechanistically so effective and powerful, it allows us to draw only one conclusion: guiding and empowering those with cancer with the knowledge and confidence they need to engage in forest bathing should be taught as a mandatory part of all robust cancer survivorship initiatives. To facilitate that, I would like to use the final section of this chapter for empowering you with everything you need to know about how and why forest bathing is so clinically significant in respect of health and healing and, even more importantly, how to actually practise it.

### The Health and Healing Benefits of Forest Bathing

The healing benefits afforded by the practice of forest bathing are unimaginably powerful, on both mind and body. These benefits are important for everyone to harness, young and old, healthy and sick, on a regular basis. In his incredible book *Last Child in the Woods*,[17] author Richard Louv makes a compelling, evidence-based argument for putting spending more time outside in nature on the same pedestal as the promotion of healthy eating, exercise and sleeping habits and stopping smoking. This is undoubtedly true. However, if we project these benefits specifically onto the arena of cancer survivorship, what we see is a veritable panacea that is clinically efficacious in the holistic management of the most common physiological and emotional side effects associated with cancer diagnosis, treatment and long-term survival. It has also been consistently shown to positively impact upon cancer-specific immune activity in powerful ways. You will find a brief overview of these benefits next.

### The Psychological and Emotional Benefits of Forest Bathing

Published evidence shows that, unsurprisingly, psychological ailments such as anxiety, stress, fear, depression, low mood and poor sleep are some of the most commonly experienced problems observed in those living with cancer.[18] The successful long-term management of these types of problems is vital if we are to thrive in the face of cancer, which is where forest bathing has an important role to play. Consider this: in one study, a single eighty-minute mindful walk in a forested environment was able to induce a clinically significant reduction in the key biochemical markers of anxiety, such as reduced adrenaline in the urine and lower levels of adiponectin in the serum.[19] This reduction in the physiological markers of anxiety was mirrored when the participants were psychologically analysed, with the results highlighting a clinically significant reduction in anxiety, fatigue and depression and a significant increase in emotional vigour and energy. It is easy to skim past these kinds of findings, but if we really meditate on them, their significance grows; here is a free, enjoyable and easy-to-perform self-care practice that is able to significantly reduce the physiological and psychological presentations of anxiety, depression and fatigue while at the same time increasing emotional vigour. Given how prevalent these types of ailments are in those living with cancer, these are powerful findings.

Or perhaps you aren't necessarily feeling anxious or depressed right now, but how about stress? Stress has become endemic in our culture and living with cancer can greatly exacerbate this. And again it appears that forest bathing gifts us a clinically proven approach for mitigating the damaging effects of stress on our body. For example, an extensive volume of published evidence shows that the practice of forest bathing is able to induce a clinically significant reduction in cortisol production.[20] This is important as lower cortisol production is the single best marker for identifying falling stress levels. So the next time you are feeling overwhelmed or stressed out, having a 'go-to' forest bathing spot to retreat to offers arguably one of the most effective, free and enjoyable remedies for managing such problems.

Another health risk that forest bathing appears to effectively mitigate is that of chronic sleep dysfunction, a problem that has been shown to impact upon more than 50 per cent of those living with cancer.[21] This is important because poorer sleep profiles have been linked to impaired immune status, increased inflammation, higher risks of fatigue, higher rates of infection, increased risk of mental health disorders and even increased mortality rates in those with cancer.[22] While harnessing the power of circadian alignment is the single most effective means of promoting optimal sleeping patterns, evidence also shows that forest bathing can significantly increase both the quality and overall quantity of sleep, in both those with and without cancer.[23] One of the potential reasons for this is that forest bathing has been shown to induce clinically significant increases in the circulating levels of the hormone serotonin,[24] which acts as a precursor to the sleep hormone melatonin. And the fact that forest bathing increases serotonin levels means the body has a greater capacity to make and use melatonin, which, as we explored previously, is vital to cultivating a good night's sleep. This may explain the positive relationship between forest bathing and sleep quality.

## The Physiological and Immunological Benefits of Forest Bathing

Some of the most powerful clinical evidence to emerge from the study of forest bathing centres upon its ability to optimise human immune activity, particularly in relation to anti-cancer defence mechanisms. What this research shows is that when we forest bathe, a clinically significant increase in the number of circulating natural killer cells (NK cells) is consistently and reliably observed.[25] This is a crucial finding because our NK cells play a foundational role within the body's collective immune response to cancer. So important is this relationship that higher NK cell status has been shown to be an independent predictor of longer survival times in those with cancer.[26] Furthermore, not only does forest bathing increase the actual number of NK cells, it has also been shown to significantly increase the release of specific anti-cancer intra-cellular proteins such as granulysin, perforin and granzymes A and B, all of which play a key role in the immunological identification and destruction of cancer cells within the tumour microenvironment. Crucially, the powerful immune-activating benefits of forest bathing have been shown to persist for up to thirty days after visiting the forest. Thus, in terms of immunological 'gain for effort', this is arguably one of the most clinically relevant and long-lasting anti-cancer immune-enhancing self-care practices that we have access to.

The magnitude of this evidence has led scientists to unpick the specific mechanisms that explain why a practice as simple as forest bathing is able to induce such profound immunological alterations. And what this research shows is that it all comes down to the celebrated phytoncides. Phytoncides are botanically labelled as volatile organic compounds (VOCs) but are better known by their colloquial name of essential oils. These essential oils have now been analysed and have been shown to possess powerful antimicrobial, insecticidal and infection-preventing properties. This makes sense because the reason trees secrete phytoncides in the first place is to create a 'force field' around them that prevents harmful bacteria, viruses and fungi from damaging them. Thus, in many ways we can think of these airborne essential oils as the tree's immune system. However, the healing potential of these phytoncides isn't exclusive to the botanical kingdom. The clinical evidence now shows that when mammals breathe in these airborne essential oils, they enter into the lungs and thenceforth into the blood. From here, they are able to exert powerful immune-stimulating and anti-inflammatory impact. The clinically significant elevations in immune status observed in the forest bathing research is down, almost exclusively, to these airborne phytoncides. This is great news for us as they provide a quick, easy and free natural medicine that we can harness in our quest to help strengthen our immune defences.

## How to Practise Forest Bathing

To effectively and evidentially harness all of the profound benefits of forest bathing, we need do nothing more than allow our conscious awareness to simply and effortlessly come to rest among our senses. For out in nature, away from the stresses and strains of the man-created world, we find the ultimate tapestry for unleashing the healing powers of tanmatra chikitsa. To do so, spend some time exploring the natural world around you. You want to find a selection of locations that deeply resonate with you because of their beauty, their ecology, their quietude and the overarching energy they emit. Try to ensure such locations are within a twenty- to thirty-minute journey of where you live so that accessing them is easy, practical and sustainable. Within these locations, try to find a specific spot that especially appeals to you. It could be a bench in a beautiful woods, an isolated tree to sit and lean against, the bank of a babbling brook or an expansive hill top with panoramic views. This is your 'sit-spot' and, if you use it properly, it will become your most trusted ally and your most revered retreat away from the world.

Come here regularly, at least once a week if possible. Sit in this sacred place and let your body become heavy. Let your mind slow as you feel the pace of modern life slip away as you align yourself with the slower rhythms of the natural world all around you. Close your eyes and turn all your attention inwards to your sense of hearing. What can you hear? What can you really hear? Narrow your world down until all that exists is the connection between you and the world around you via the portal of your auditory nerves. Can you hear the wind rustling the branches in the trees above you? Can you hear the deeply calming sound of birdsong? Can you hear insects rummaging in the leaf litter beneath your feet? Move beyond just listening to these sounds and rather try to become them as they occupy the entire sphere of your awareness, and stay in this awareness for as long as feels right for you.

Then, still keeping your eyes closed, allow your laser-focused auditory attention to dissipate and switch instead to the olfactory nerves in your nose and the healing sense of smell. Breathe in deeply and slowly through your nose; what can you smell? The heady scent of pine oils, the earthy smell of leaf litter, the unmistakable aroma of tree blossom? Perhaps turn your head one way and then the other to connect with these smells in a more powerful way. Again, deeply connect with these healing aromas. If you are in a forest, bring your conscious awareness to the fact that, as you breathe in the airborne phytocides all around you, these will go on to activate your anti-cancer immunity in powerful and observable ways. Revere these scents as you breathe them in, acknowledging the proactive role you are playing in harnessing the powers of sensory healing in your quest to become exceptional. Feel these scents galvanising and energising you.

Slowly open your eyes and bring your awareness to your visual sense. What vistas open up in front of you that made you choose this place specifically? Why do you love this spot, visually speaking? Perhaps shift your gaze skywards and watch the meditative sway of the treetops above you as they dance in the wind. Lose yourself in the transient beauty of autumnal leaves as they gently fall to earth. Feel your heart overflow with joy as you watch the aerial gymnastics of a squirrel in a neighbouring tree. Move beyond simply watching and rather try to become that which you observe. If a cherry tree in full blossom captivates you, focus on those blossoms to such a degree that, for a few brief minutes, nothing but those blossoms exists in your sensory awareness.

This losing of oneself in the majesty of the senses is exactly what tanmatra chikitsa is all about as a healing modality. If you wanted to, and the weather is fine, you could perhaps remove your shoes and socks and connect your feet directly to the earth to engage the kinaesthetic sense of touch. And then when you feel saturated and satisfied with the healing capacity your sit-spot has gifted you, perhaps you might, with a heart filled with gratitude, carefully unpack your backpack. From this you might pour yourself a steaming cup of aromatic coffee or herbal tea.

From personal experience, I can tell you that sitting in silence, surrounded by the majesty of the natural world, mindfully drinking a steaming cup of fresh coffee with your face turned to the sun is perhaps one of the most life-affirming things I have ever done. I can recall certain instances where I achieved an almost transcendent state doing this and I was filled with such an outpouring of joy that I felt truly euphoric. The level of healing that accompanies these types of responses is unimaginably powerful and almost impossible to quantify. But it works. And then perhaps, as you sip your coffee, you notice a pleasant stirring of hunger and, again with mindful gratitude, you pull from your daypack a simple picnic of tasty and fulfilling anti-cancer foods. As you eat, you engage your final sense – taste – as you acknowledge the healing mechanisms these foods mobilise.

After a certain period of time, you will feel ready (but often reluctant!) to leave this place, and when you do so, you will not be walking away from your sit-spot in the same body that you arrived in; your entire physiology and biochemistry, not to mention your mood and emotions, will have altered in powerful ways towards the direction of healing. And this level of healing is discernible if you consciously focus on how you actually feel in your body and mind after such experiences. This is why Ayurveda places such emphasis on the activation of sensory healing via the framework of tanmatra chikitsa and why we all should too.

##  Chapter Affirmations for My Journey to Becoming Exceptional

1. I consciously acknowledge the power of my senses to induce transformative levels of healing in my body and mind.
2. I recognise the Ayurvedic practice of tanmatra chikitsa as an all-encompassing framework for harnessing and unleashing the power of sensory healing in my daily life.
3. I commit to accessing my sensory healing pathways every day, using the method that feels right for me on that specific day.
4. I consciously acknowledge the transformative and evidence-based anti-cancer impacts of forest bathing, and I commit to seeking out and using a nature sit-spot as often as I comfortably and feasibly can.
5. **Summary Affirmation:** Each and every day I will harness and unleash the powerful healing responses initiated via sensory healing as I powerfully and purposefully progress along the path of becoming exceptional.

# CHAPTER TEN

# Putting Out the Fires

## *Managing the Side Effects of Conventional Cancer Treatments*

> *I believe that for every ailment known to man, God has created a plant that will heal it.*
> VANNOY GENTLES FITE, *Essential Oils for Healing*

In the quest to become exceptional in the face of cancer, a truly integrative approach to treatment is the best one. This is an approach that sees us harnessing all of the benefits afforded by conventional cancer medicine while at the same time integrating safe and evidence-based natural approaches alongside these, such as those explored and advocated in this book. Doing so allows us to harness the benefits and advantages of both in a mutually supportive and harmonious way. This is particularly true in light of the increasing development of exciting new anti-cancer drugs. For example, the huge progress being made within the field of immunotherapy shows real promise in the context of extending survival times in those with cancer, in some cases by more than 15 per cent.[1] Similarly, the release in early 2024 of a new classification of antibody drug called Daratumumab has had a tremendous impact upon improving both quality of life and survival times in those with certain types of cancer.[2] It appears that we are currently entering into an exciting new era of cancer medicine that offers an ever-increasing sense of hope and optimism. And this is to be applauded.

However, all pharmacological cancer treatments come with a price and that price is their side-effect profile. These side effects span the full spectrum of severity, ranging from relatively minor annoyances all the way through to severe and often debilitating symptomology. Fortunately, these types of side effects are usually very well managed within conventional care. That said, it is always useful

> **A Note of Caution**
> As stressed in chapter 7, it is important to re-emphasise that you must never start taking a new herbal medicine or supplement during active cancer treatment without the explicit consent of your consultant to ensure there is no risk of drug – herb interaction.

and empowering to have access to an additional toolbox of safe and clinically proven natural options that can be used alongside their conventional counterparts to help in the holistic management of any such side effects or symptoms.

Over the years, I have seen these types of natural remedies make a significant positive impact on the overall quality of life of those progressing through cancer treatment and I wholeheartedly recommend them to you. The aim of this chapter is to explore a selection of safe, gentle and proven natural remedies for the adjunct management of the most common side effects experienced by those going through chemotherapy and radiotherapy treatment.

## Managing Common Chemotherapy- and Radiotherapy-Induced Side Effects

### 1. Fatigue

Of the most commonly listed cancer treatment-induced side effects, fatigue and exhaustion are arguably the most common, with evidence suggesting a prevalence rate of between 60 per cent and 90 per cent.[3] Such problems can have a debilitating impact upon overall quality of life and it is therefore important that steps are taken to alleviate the severity of the fatigue experienced. Here are some simple and proven suggestions for doing so.

**Walking/Aerobic Exercise**

As counter-intuitive as it may sound, movement is arguably one of the simplest and most effective remedies for reducing the severity of treatment-induced fatigue.[4] For example, in women with breast cancer going though chemotherapeutic treatment, taking part in a twelve-week walking intervention was able to significantly reduce the severity of fatigue experienced in comparison to a matched group not engaging in the walking intervention.[5] Similar results have been observed in many other cancer cohorts, the result of which is that most national health services, including the UK's National Health Service, recommend the use of gentle aerobic exercise as a vital aspect of staying well during cancer treatment.

It is impossible to be prescriptive with regard to the volume and intensity of exercise undertaken, as this will vary greatly depending upon your individual circumstances. The best advice is to listen to your body and ensure that you always do a little less than you think you can. This is because if you push too hard, exercise can exacerbate rather than alleviate fatigue-based symptoms. So, listen to your body and try to exercise or move your body as often as you comfortably can, be that a gentle walk, a little gardening, simple housework or a slow bike ride. Seeking the advice of a suitably qualified exercise professional is also greatly recommended so that a fully individualised exercise plan can be formulated.

## Synbiotics

The impact of the gut microbiome on the management of cancer treatment side effects, including fatigue, has shot into the research spotlight in recent years. The collective weight of evidence from this research suggests real promise in the use of prebiotics and probiotics in the effective management of fatigue. In particular, the use of synbiotic supplements – which are a combination of prebiotics and probiotics in one single supplement – appears to be especially effective. For example, in a cohort of women with breast cancer going through chemotherapy, the use of a daily synbiotic supplement was able to induce a clinically significant reduction in the severity of fatigue while also reducing the symptoms of nausea, vomiting and diarrhoea.[6] Given this, I would strongly encourage you to explore the use of synbiotic supplements with your clinical care team as a means of supporting improved energy and vitality during treatment. See Prebiotic, Probiotic and Synbiotic Supplements in appendix 3 (page 228) for details of my recommended synbiotic supplier.

## Astragalus

A third and final natural treatment that excels in the management of cancer-related fatigue is the famous Eastern herb astragalus. You will recall that in chapter 7 we explored the powerful anti-cancer impacts and mechanisms of astragalus in a more general capacity. However, above and beyond this, several clinical studies have been published that have specifically revealed that astragalus is able to induce clinically significant reductions in the severity of fatigue in those going through cancer treatment.[7] And while it is important to highlight that in some cases the astragalus was administered intravenously as isolated extracts of the herb (as opposed to using the pure, whole herb), the available evidence strongly suggests that the use of astragalus in pure form may significantly reduce the degree of fatigue experienced. I would recommend exploring the use of this herb with your clinical care team.

## 2. Nausea and Vomiting

According to the latest statistics, the National Cancer Institute in the US estimates that up to 80 per cent of those going through cancer treatment experience nausea and vomiting.[8] These are significant symptoms that not only greatly reduce daily quality of life but also make it very hard to ensure the sufficient daily intake of the required anti-cancer foods we previously explored. Fortunately, anti-emetic drugs are typically very effective at reducing the severity and prevalence of treatment-induced nausea and vomiting these days. However, even with such treatment, a chronic, lingering sense of nausea often remains, which can be unpleasant to live with. To help combat this, there are a selection of tried-and-tested natural remedies that offer real potential in further mitigating the severity and prevalence of nausea and vomiting in those progressing through cancer treatment. Some of the most important of these are explored below:

### Ginger

A time-tested and revered medicine from within the Ayurvedic tradition, ginger has been pressed into service as a herbal anti-emetic for millennia. The clinical evidence supports this notion, identifying a selection of chemicals found within ginger, such as 6-shogaol, 6-gingerol and zingerone, that are able to modify the biochemical mechanisms within the gastrointestinal tract and help to suppress nausea and vomiting.[9] Also of great interest is the fact that ginger has shown promising results in the specific management of chemotherapy- and radiotherapy-induced nausea. For example, in a large cohort of close to six hundred cancer patients going through chemotherapy, it was observed that those taking ginger supplements experienced a clinically significant reduction in nausea and vomiting in comparison to those taking a placebo.[10] To harness these benefits, clinical guidelines advocate the importance of starting ginger treatment before chemotherapy is administered to maximise the benefits obtained.[11] To use ginger in this way, simply mix one teaspoon of freshly grated ginger, or half a teaspoon of dried ground ginger, into a cup and pour over boiling water, leave to cool and then drink as a herbal tea. Aim to drink two to three cups per day.

## Essential Oils

Another great option for the holistic management of nausea and vomiting is the use of essential oils. As we explored in the previous chapter, essential oils are able to impart powerful responses in the physiological workings of the body via the olfactory nerves. The published research shows that through doing so, essential oils may be of real help to those experiencing cancer treatment-induced nausea and vomiting. A very well-designed study from the US looked at the use of peppermint essential oil as a treatment for reducing nausea in those going through chemotherapy. The results showed that in the cohort of over 70 patients taking part in the study, the use of peppermint oil on a cool damp washcloth placed on the neck was effective in relieving nausea compared to using a cool damp washcloth alone.[12]

Similarly, a recent meta-analysis (which represents the highest standard of clinical evidence) exploring the use of essential oils in the management of cancer-treatment nausea and vomiting revealed that out of the nine independent studies analysed, seven showed a clinically significant reduction in the severity of the nausea and vomiting symptoms experienced. These results were obtained from the use of ginger, chamomile, cardamom and peppermint essential oils.[13] The use of an essential oil diffuser is arguably the simplest way of harnessing these benefits. These heat and disperse essential oils via steam and are incredibly effective as they provide a constant and steady supply of essential oil molecules into the air all around you. Alternatively, the essential oil can be added to a cool, damp washcloth and placed on the back of the neck, as described above.

## Acupressure

Acupressure uses the application of pressure to the energy centres of the body. On the wrist there is a famous acupressure point called Neiguan (nay-gwann), which is now clinically proven to alleviate the nausea and vomiting associated with travel sickness when stimulated via the use of wrist travel bands. However, these gains appear to transfer to the alleviation of cancer treatment-induced nausea and vomiting too. For example, a clinical study observed that in individuals going through chemotherapy, those wearing travel bands that stimulated the Neiguan point experienced a clinically significant reduction in nausea, vomiting and retching occurrence in comparison to those receiving placebo treatment.[14] Wrist travel bands such as these are readily available from any good chemist or online retailers.

## 3. Oral Mouth Ulcers/Mucositis

As an incredibly common side effect of both chemotherapy and radiotherapy, mucositis (oral inflammation) and mouth ulcers are painful conditions that can greatly reduce quality of life. Eating and drinking becomes difficult and painful, and in severe cases largely impossible, and even talking can be unpleasant. It is vital that these types of problems are effectively managed. Fortunately, there are lots of conventional treatments that can be used to help both prevent and treat mucositis, including pain killers, anaesthetic mouthwashes, anti-inflammatories and ice therapy. In addition to these approaches, there are a selection of incredibly helpful natural treatments that can really help to further alleviate the distressing symptoms associated with mucositis. These include:

### Raw Honey

Arguably the most important natural remedy to implement before and during chemotherapy and radiotherapy treatment to help prevent and manage the severity of mucositis is raw honey therapy. In Ayurvedic medicine, raw honey has been used as a topical salve to aid healing and reduce pain and inflammation for millennia. This use is validated by the published evidence, which has identified honey as being a clinically effective treatment for tissue healing, burns, wounds, ulcers and topical inflammation.[15] Mechanistically, this is because honey has been shown to effectively stimulate the increased release of cytokines, which are proteins that play an instrumental role in inflammation regulation and tissue healing.[16] Additionally, the high concentrations of vitamins, enzymes and antibacterial agents found in honey further support its infection-preventing and wound-healing properties. In light of these benefits, several studies have clinically tested the use of honey as a remedy for preventing and treating cancer treatment-induced oral mucositis. These studies have shown that honey was able to reduce the onset of moderate to severe mucositis by up to 75 per cent.[17] Honey treatment helped to prevent the development of intolerable levels of mucositis too, while also supporting faster healing times.[18]

**Using Honey Treatment:** As a preventative before starting chemotherapy or radiotherapy treatment, simply place 1 teaspoon of raw (non-heated) honey into your mouth and swish this all around your oral cavity so that it coats the inside of the cheeks, tongue, back of the throat and the roof of the mouth before spitting it out. Repeat this three times daily for ten days before treatment begins. This process can be repeated every three hours during treatment to help manage any side effects that occur.

### Sage, Thyme and Peppermint Mouth Rinse
In addition to the use of raw honey, herbal mouth rinses using sage, thyme and peppermint have shown clinical efficacy in reducing the prevalence of mucositis in those receiving chemotherapy. These benefits were believed to be due to the proven antiseptic and anti-inflammatory properties inherent within these herbs.[19] While this study used a hydrosol (a form of herbal water) to deliver these herbs, a simple herbal tea would be just as effective.

To make, simply add 1 teaspoon each of dried sage, thyme and peppermint to a cup and pour over boiling water. Leave to steep until cool and then strain out the herbs. To use, swish this cooled herbal tea gently around the mouth for one to two minutes before spitting out the liquid (do not swallow it). Repeat every two to three hours. If using fresh herbs, increase the dose to 2 teaspoons of each herb as opposed to the 1 teaspoon listed above.

## 5. Nerve Pain/Neuropathy
Both chemotherapy and radiotherapy treatments can damage nerve tissue, leading to the chronic nerve pain that is a common side effect of these types of treatments. In most instances these problems gradually improve over time once treatment has ended. However, there is much that can be done to alleviate the severity of pain experienced while also speeding up recovery time. Here are some top natural remedies to explore in this capacity:

## Yoga

As the sister science of Ayurveda, yoga offers profound health-giving benefits that positively impact upon the workings of every cell and organ system in the body. Yoga has a vital role to play in the cultivation of optimal health when living with and surviving cancer. And while a full treatise on the use of yoga in the context of cancer survivorship is beyond the scope of this book, it is worth highlighting the positive impact it has been shown to have upon cancer treatment-induced nerve pain. For example, in a cohort of breast and gynaecological cancer patients experiencing moderate to severe nerve pain, undertaking an eight-week yoga intervention resulted in a clinically significant reduction in the severity and prevalence of the nerve pain experienced in comparison to those not receiving the yoga intervention.[20] I strongly recommend the exploration of yoga therapy as an adjunct treatment for nerve pain and that you seek the advice of a qualified and experienced yoga teacher to facilitate this in a safe and individualised manner.

## Capsaicin Patches

Capsaicin is a naturally occurring compound found in chilli peppers that is responsible for the heating sensation experienced when we eat them. Capsaicin is a potent pain killer that works to blocks the biochemical messengers of pain from our nerve cells. It has been shown to possess clinical efficacy in reducing the prevalence and severity of peripheral nerve pain, irrespective of the cause.[21] This includes the effective management of cancer treatment-induced nerve pain. For example, an incredibly well-designed clinical trial published in 2023 revealed that the use of topical capsaicin patches was able to induce a clinically significant reduction in cancer treatment-induced nerve pain in a cohort of female cancer patients going through chemotherapeutic treatment.[22] So effective is the pain-killing capacity of topical capsaicin patches that the European Society for Medical Oncology (ESMO) lists high-concentration capsaicin patches as their recommended second-line treatment for nerve pain subsequent to the use of conventional pharmacological treatments.[23] Topical capsaicin patches are available in both prescription and over-the-counter formats, so please discuss their use with your clinical care team so that the options for your individual case can be explored and the best one decided upon.

## 6. Muscle Aches and Pains

In the same way that chemotherapy and radiotherapy can damage nerve cells, they can also damage muscle tissue. This in turn leads to the common types of muscle aches and pains that are so prevalent in those receiving such treatments. If you are suffering with any such problems, here are some excellent natural remedies to try:

### Mahanarayan Oil

A true hidden gem, Mahanarayan oil is Ayurveda's most revered topical treatment for the management of all types of muscle aches and pains. Having prescribed this remarkable oil to thousands of people suffering with muscle pain over the years, it is hard for me to over-emphasise the impacts it can have. Made up of over twenty different anti-inflammatory, anti-spasmodic and analgesic herbal medicines, all macerated into a concentrated herbal oil, it really can impart almost miraculous healing responses. To use, simply warm a few tablespoons of the oil over a flame (never in the microwave as this will destroy the active herbal constituents) and simply massage slowly and deeply into the areas of pain. Alternatively, use this oil for your morning self-massage as described in Ayurvedic Oil Massage: Self-Abhyanga on page 152 in chapter 8. Details of my recommended suppliers of authentic Mahanarayan oil are listed under Ayurvedic Body and Massage Oils in appendix 3 (page 228).

### Epsom Salt Baths

Another fantastic, centuries-old natural remedy for alleviating muscular aches and pains is to take an Epsom salt bath. Slipping into a beautiful, hot Epsom salt bath very often sees us re-emerge feeling revitalised, relaxed and soothed. Thus, if you are suffering with muscle or body aches, this is a fantastically relaxing natural remedy to try. Epsom salt is readily available from any good health food shop or chemist. To use, please follow the manufacturer's instructions.

## 7. Radiotherapy-Induced Skin, Mouth and Throat Discomfort

Radiotherapy can cause significant pain and burning to the surface of the skin around which it is administered. When this treatment is delivered in the management of head and neck cancers, it can cause burning and ulceration in the mouth and throat that can make eating, drinking and even talking difficult. There are an increasing number of effective conventional treatments for lessening the incidence and severity of such problems but, if additional help is needed, the following remedies will be of help:

### Raw Honey

As discussed previously, honey is a tremendously effective remedy for the management of mucositis in the mouth caused by both chemotherapy and radiotherapy. Thus, if there are any signs of burning, trauma or inflammation in the mouth or throat as a specific result of radiotherapy treatment, please follow the previous advice on the use of honey to help prevent and manage such problems.

### Topical Aloe Vera

Another brilliant option for alleviating radiotherapy-induced skin burns and soreness is the use of topical aloe vera. Many of us have turned to this amazing herbal medicine to soothe sunburn and as an after-sun remedy because of its inherently cooling, repairing and anti-inflammatory properties. In the same way, we can also turn to aloe vera as a proven and effective remedy in the topical management of skin discomfort caused by radiotherapy. Indeed, several published clinical studies have observed that that topical application of aloe vera was able to induce clinically significant reductions in the severity of both chemotherapy- and radiotherapy-induced skin symptoms in comparison to the use of soap, placebos or phospholipid cream.[24] To harness these benefits, simply purchase a top-quality, pure aloe vera gel and massage this gently onto the skin several times a day before and after treatment.

## 8. Anxiety

Unsurprisingly, anxiety is endemic in those living with cancer and can greatly reduce overall quality of life. While there are a wide range of conventional pharmaceutical treatments that offer real efficacy in the management of anxiety, natural options can also work wonderfully well, especially in situations where one wants to avoid conventional treatments and the side effects that often accompany them. Here are some great options for doing so.

### Herbal Infusions

Hot herbal teas, made using a variety of calming anti-anxiety herbs, can work wonders in reducing the severity of anxiety. There are a wide variety of herbs that are proven in this capacity, some of the most effective of which include rosemary, lavender, tulsi, thyme, passionflower, peppermint and lemon balm. Many of these herbs can be sourced as pre-prepared teabags from any good health food shop or online retailer. Alternatively, you can very easily source these herbs in loose, dried form from online herb dispensaries. If using the former, simply aim to drink two to three cups a day. If using the latter, simply add one teaspoon of the herbs you are using into a cup, pour over boiling water and leave to infuse for ten minutes before straining and drinking. Aim to have two to three cups a day.

## Herbal Baths

The use of hot herbal baths is a fantastic way of melting away stress, anxiety and tension and elevating mood. Not only are baths in and of themselves incredibly calming, the addition of anti-anxiety herbs greatly enhances the clinical gains obtained. Herbal baths are made by pouring strong herbal infusions into a warm/hot bath (as you prefer) and mixing it thoroughly into the entire bath volume. Once in the bath, the active chemical constituents of the herbs are absorbed into the body trans-dermally (through the skin), entering the bloodstream and nervous system, from where they impart their therapeutic impacts. The chemical constituents of the herbs also enter into the body via the herbal steam given off by the hot bath water. This herbal steam is breathed in through the nose and into the lungs, where they are again absorbed into the bloodstream. As the skin is the largest organ of the body, and given that around 90 per cent of the skin surface area is immersed in the herbal bath water, the volume of active chemical constituents entering into the body via herbal baths is incredibly high, making this a very gentle yet powerful means of administering herbal medicines.

### HOW TO MAKE HERBAL BATHS

1. First, make a strong herbal infusion by placing 3–4 tablespoons of your dried herbs into a large mixing bowl. Great options include rosemary, lavender, tulsi, thyme, lime flowers, passionflower, peppermint or lemon balm.
2. Pour over a pint of boiling water and leave to infuse for at least fifteen minutes but ideally longer. A great approach is to make the infusion in the morning and place a lid over the top of the bowl to ensure the vapours don't escape. Leave it to infuse all day so that it is ready to use in the evening.

3. Once the infusion is ready, strain it through a sieve into a bowl and then pour the liquid infusion into a deep, hot bath.
4. Thoroughly mix the infusion into the bathwater so that it is evenly dispersed. Aim to remain in the bath for fifteen to twenty minutes.

**The Natural World**

Quiet, contemplative time spent in the natural world is, for me, arguably the most effective way of dialling down anxiety and stress and increasing emotional vitality. In particular, the practice of forest bathing has, in clinical trials, been proven to be effective at significantly reducing the severity and prevalence of stress, anxiety and depression. See Forest Bathing: The Ultimate Cancer-Specific Sensory Experience on page 180 to remind yourself of how to harness these benefits.

## Seeking Additional Support

In addition to the specific advice provided above, there is so much help and support available with regard to helping you better manage any side effects or symptoms you are experiencing. This help can and should firstly come from within your conventional care pathways, such as the Macmillan support services offered free of charge within the cancer care framework in Britain. In addition to this in-house support, there is a huge variety of options for help and support outside of it. Learning how to best access and utilise this support is an integral aspect of a truly robust cancer survivorship protocol. This is a hugely empowering process that allows us to build a powerful and fully integrative support system around ourselves; when we need extra help, support or advice around managing any aspect of cancer or its treatment, we immediately know where to turn. This then allows us to act quickly and effectively to proactively address any symptoms, problems or concerns we have. The building of a trusted multi-disciplinary support network in this way is a practice that is hugely beneficial and one that I can't advocate enough. Over many years of helping people with this process, I have found it is best to break this down into three key areas, as explored below.

### One-to-One Support

In my opinion, building a multi-disciplinary team of qualified healthcare professionals around you is a prerequisite for thriving in the face of cancer. Living with cancer is a fluid and dynamic process; physical and emotional problems ebb and flow in different ways, at different times and with varying degrees of severity. There is no magic bullet that is perfectly suited to managing this dynamism. For example, you may find that a counsellor or psychotherapist is more effective at managing stress and fear than an acupuncturist. However, you may find that your acupuncturist is more effective at managing pain and insomnia. Similarly, you may find a medical herbalist gives you the confidence that you need to use herbal medicines properly, while your homeopath works best to improve your mood and emotional vitality. The list goes on, but the point remains; there exists a huge array of complementary medical support resources that all excel in different ways. The more of these you have access to, the more likely you are to find success in managing and overcoming problems, be they in mind or body, when they occur. To enable this, I would highly recommend that you look into building a team of such experts around yourself. This could incorporate practitioners from a diverse array of fields, including reiki, acupuncture, homeopathy, massage therapy, Ayurveda, herbal medicine, personal trainers, counsellors and psychotherapists. Many of these practitioners have a particular interest in supporting those with cancer. To find them, integrative cancer charities are the best place to start as they have a designated directory of fully qualified and experienced experts.

## Integrative Cancer Charities

Charities that advocate the use of evidence-based integrative medicine within the arena of cancer are changing the face of oncology in many countries, particularly in Britain. They act as the primary sounding board and first port of call for those with cancer who are looking to empower themselves with all of the knowledge, support and resources they require in their quest to maximise their survivorship. The specific aims and scope of such charities vary considerably but their overarching focus is the same: the proactive empowerment and inspiration of those living with cancer to reach for a new reality with respect to their diagnosis.

To start you off on the road to exploring different service providers, I would strongly recommend Yes to Life as a great launching point. This incredible charity, based in the UK, provides a huge array of free, online resources, ranging from support groups and guided self-care sessions to international directories of other integrative cancer charitable and commercial service providers. They also man a free telephone support service that allows you to talk to a trained professional who can listen, provide advice and signpost you to relevant sources of support specific to any issues or problems you may be experiencing. You can find out more and explore their services at www.yestolife.org.uk.

### Online Cancer Support Forums

Last but not least is the help and support offered by online cancer support forums. These are usually cancer-site specific (that is, the forums are for individuals with a specific type of cancer, such as liver or breast cancer) and allow for an incredibly inspiring level of peer support. Regularly connecting with others who are living with and managing the same type of cancer as you comes with a wealth of benefits. It allows for the sharing of fears and concerns, discussions around treatments, strategies for coping with side effects, the sharing of resources and the provision of emotional support and so much else. There is a huge array of both in-person and online cancer-specific support services available depending on your specific geographical location. Your designated cancer nurse will be best placed to signpost you towards the best group to approach and I can't recommend doing so enough.

##  Chapter Affirmations for My Journey to Becoming Exceptional

1. I will proactively research the very best natural remedies that will maximise my ability to effectively manage any symptoms or side effects I experience.
2. I acknowledge that living with ineffectively managed side effects is not acceptable and I will seek the very best advice from my conventional care team to overcome this.
3. In addition to this, I will build a powerful multi-disciplinary team of qualified and experienced complementary health professionals around me that I can call upon when symptoms or side effects occur.
4. I will seek out the very best integrative, charitable and peer-to-peer support to allow me to increasingly reinforce the effectiveness of my cancer survivorship protocol.
5. **Summary Affirmation:** Each and every day I commit to pressing into service the full might of integrative medicine as I powerfully and purposefully progress along the path of becoming exceptional.

## CHAPTER ELEVEN

# Bringing It All Together
## *The 5-Step Plan*

> *Here's to the crazy ones. The misfits. The rebels. The troublemakers. The round pegs in the square holes. The ones who see things differently. They're not fond of rules. And they have no respect for the status quo ... And while some may see them as the crazy ones, we see genius. Because the people who are crazy enough to think they can change the world, are the ones who do.*
>
> APPLE, 'Think Different'

When Steve Jobs spoke these beautifully moving but challenging words, he was referring to the people who were shaking up and disrupting the otherwise stagnant world of digital technology. More than any other quote I have ever read, it exemplifies in an unparalleled way the exact type of outlook that exceptional cancer patients proactively cultivate. To have the courage and inner fortitude to choose a different reality in the face of cancer, particularly when that reality flies in the face of an all-pervading sense of hopelessness and fatalism, requires of us an urgent need to see things differently. It also requires us to completely disrespect the status quo of cancer statistics and doom-laden prognoses. How could it be otherwise? If Janet, whom we met in the introduction, or Roger Bannister, who first broke the four-minute mile, had not proactively chosen to see things differently and challenge the status quo of their situation, it is highly unlikely that they would have realised exceptionality.

Over the last fifteen years, I have had the immense privilege of meeting so many people living with cancer who have gone on to become exceptional. And when I do so, I always see genius. I see round pegs who refused to fit into the square holes of their prognoses. I see rebels who defiantly mutineered against the all-pervading hopelessness of their situation. Like Steve Jobs, I also recognise a little craziness in them. Because I think, at least initially, rebelling in this way does require a healthy dose of craziness. But it is not blind, lost or uninformed craziness. It is empowered craziness. It's focused, it's fearless and it is relentless.

Those who become exceptional intuitively realise that to become different they ultimately have to do different. In other words, if they are to break from the crowd and thrive in the face of cancer, they have to do things that the majority of those with cancer don't or won't do. That is not to imply any sense of judgment whatsoever. It simply means that to become exceptional, the concept of the exceptional must saturate our behaviours, actions, thoughts, beliefs and attitudes in their entirety. It can be no other way; exceptionality is always forged upon the anvil of our actions.

All the way through this book, we have been exploring some of the most important of these actions. We have covered an eclectic array of topics that span every facet of our daily lives from the moment we wake up to the time we go to bed; the foods we eat, the routines we follow, the self-care practices we adopt, the herbs we take, the mindsets we cultivate and so much more. All of these behaviours are advocated because of the compelling published evidence that highlights the positive impact they can have upon the optimisation of health when living with cancer. That much is clear. But to leave it there is to miss the bigger picture. So, as we move to concluding this book, we have to finish where we started. In chapter 2, we explored the infinite potential for healing that exists as an inherent part of the human body. We also explored examples of how profound this healing mechanism is. But we shouldn't think of exceptional healing as being the exclusive domain of a lucky few who have been blessed with the mechanisms for facilitating it.

Exceptional healing is available to all of us, all of the time. In fact, and somewhat paradoxically, I would go as far as to say that exceptional healing isn't exceptional at all. Rather, it is the normal healing potential of the body that is only activated exceptionally rarely. We can sometimes lose sight of this fact. We can lose sight of the sheer mystery of the human body and its infinite capacity for self-regulation. The body's default setting is always to move towards healing and away from disease. Even in the face of the most advanced and overwhelming pathological states there exists the opportunity for this. The publication in leading medical journals of incredibly inspiring clinical case studies of people living with some of the most advanced and aggressive forms of cancer who go on to become exceptional shows just how profound this healing potential is. The fact that it is increasingly being recognised and acknowledged in the arena of conventional medicine is hugely encouraging.

As we have previously explored, what allows for these types of exceptional healing responses is the fact that the body is dynamic. It is constantly rebuilding and recreating itself in an impossibly complex and creative way. What this means for us at the practical level is that at any given point in time we can consciously choose to act in a way that presses this dynamism into the service of creating the new type of body we desire. The body you inhabit right now, as you sit reading this book, is not the body you will possess this time tomorrow, this time next week or this time next year. It simply isn't. You have the ability to inform, in any given second, whether your body moves towards dynamic regeneration or towards stagnant atrophy. You don't have to buy into, or subscribe to, the status quo that states that the body or illness you currently have is the one you will always have. It all comes down to potential and choice. If you choose, in an empowered way, to nourish your body with the raw materials that contain the potential to induce healing, the inner intelligence that resides in every cell of your body will use that raw potential to create transformation. Not sometimes, possibly or occasionally. It will do it all of the time, in every second of every day.

Take, as a singular example, something as seemingly basic as an atom of oxygen. This one individual atom, floating randomly past you in a specific moment of time, seemingly has no bearing upon you as a person or upon your health, healing potential or survival. That is until you take an in-breath and it flows into your lungs. From here, it will pass through your respiratory membranes and enter into your blood, whence it will attach to a molecule of haemoglobin. At this point in time, a miracle occurs that is unparalleled in impact; that random oxygen atom that had no relevance to you before you breathed it in has now physically and tangibly become you. It has become part of the very fabric of your body. That atom of oxygen, and trillions of others, will go on to nourish and sustain the life and healing potential of every single cell in your body, without which you would cease to exist. So, too, with every mouthful of food you eat, every sight you see, every molecule of water you drink, every uplifting poem you read, every evocative smell you experience, every goal you visualise, every herbal medicine you consume and every other healing practice you adopt. The healing potential found in these things doesn't simply nourish you, it becomes you.

This is an act of creation that is unrivalled in breadth and unmatched in impact. For in consciously controlling what raw material you put into your body, you have the unique ability to rebuild it in any way you desire. If you desire stronger and more capable anti-cancer immune activity, you can choose to provide your body with the raw materials it needs to facilitate this. If you desire a life lived with more meaning, purpose and passion, you can choose to saturate your senses with activities that provide this.

At the base level, this dynamic conversion of the raw material of potential into a tangible and quantitative healing response is regulated by the inherent inner intelligence found within the body. Ayurveda labels this as the doshas. When the doshas are unbalanced, the dynamic healing potential of the body is suppressed and this potential for healing remains just that. But when the doshas are balanced and working harmoniously, this healing dynamism is fully unleashed in the most powerful of ways, allowing the potential to be actualised. It is for this reason that the removal of vikruti – the disease-forming dust on the hard wooden surface of prakruti that we learned about on page 16 in Ayurveda: The Science of Optimal Living – is of such importance.

All of the practices and techniques explored in this book are aimed at removing vikruti and continually restoring balance to the doshas in this way. But they do so from a place of optimal duality. For example, regular meditation practice does afford unequivocal health benefits at the physical and mental level to those living with cancer. The clinical published research clearly supports this. But that is just one side of the coin. On the other side – the Ayurvedic side – we acknowledge the powerful ability of meditation to harmonise the workings of the doshas so as to fully optimise their healing potential. Or again, the Western clinical evidence has revealed that going to bed at the correct time to support optimal sleep profiles is a vital component of cancer survivorship. Ayurveda also recognises this, not just as a means of supporting optimal sleep but also as a means of maintaining optimal balance among the doshas so as to best unleash their healing dynamism.

The list goes on but the point remains; every second of every day our body's default setting is to move towards healing and self-preservation. It will move mountains to facilitate this but only if it is given the tools to do so. The aim of this book has ultimately been the provision of these tools. And it has been to provide them in a way that combines the very best of Western evidence-based cancer survivorship research along with the practices and approaches of

Ayurveda. But as we said previously, if you are going to break from the crowd and become exceptional you have to be prepared to do what others won't. In other words, you have to actually implement the tools and techniques covered in the previous chapters. Because for these practices to work, they have to be applied on a long-term basis. To be applied on a long-term basis they need to be sustainable. And to be sustainable, they need to be easy and effortless to adopt and comply with on an ongoing basis. Having worked on and implemented clinical trials looking at long-term health behaviour change in this way – particularly in those with cancer – I can say with absolute certainty that the best way of doing so is to harness the power of a practice called *kaizen*.

Kaizen relates to the process of initiating and sustaining positive behavioural change by way of small, progressive and continual improvement that over time amounts to transformational levels of change. The best available behavioural change research shows that using this approach maximises our chances of long-term success because the changes facing us don't appear too daunting or insurmountable. Overhauling our entire way of life overnight is doomed to failure because the mountain appears too big for us to climb in one go. Using every ounce of our will power, we might comply for a week or two, but ultimately the task appears too overwhelming and we begin to slip with our practices, our motivation drops and we ultimately fail before we even really begin. You may have seen this play out in your own life if you have ever set a New Year's resolution. You set off with the very best of intentions, but in just a few short weeks or months, the change you were so motivated to see is not realised.

But with kaizen, we can prevent this. By looking at the ultimate goal and end point – thriving in the face of cancer – and selecting just one practice to adopt that moves you a little closer to realising that goal, you feel that practically speaking you will be able to actually embed this one small change on a sustainable long-term basis. As you begin to do so, you experience a genuine sense of achievement, which in turn engenders increased motivation to continue. This then further embeds your sense of success. Once this single small change has been effortlessly adopted into your daily life in a way that is self-fulfilling and sustainable, you then pick another small change to focus on while keeping the previous one running. And then you repeat the process until this second practice also becomes habitual. You then continue to repeat this process until *all* of the changes you wish to make have been progressively built into your daily or weekly routine in a practical and sustainable way.

When teaching the concept of kaizen to others, I find the analogy of Hercules and the bull a really helpful one. Arguably the most famous of all the ancient Greek heroes, Hercules was celebrated for his super-human strength. This was a strength that allowed him to lift a fully grown bull above his head, a feat that was famed across the Greek empire and one that was regarded as the epitome of human potential. But what no one except Hercules and his mentor knew was that his ability to lift the bull was not down to God-given super-human strength but rather strategy. More specifically, it was due to kaizen. For what allowed him to achieve this supposedly impossible feat was that from when the bull was born, he would pick it up and lift it above his head once a day. In this way the small, negligible daily increments in weight gain in the bull were matched by an equally small daily increase in Hercules' strength. As the bull grew heavier, Hercules grew stronger until such a point that he was able to pick up a fully grown bull. If Hercules, or any other man, had tried to do so without the use of a progressive approach such as this, it would have been impossible. But by using the practice of kaizen it became possible. Hercules became exceptional not down to 'genetic luck' but by small daily progression.

So, too, with us when it comes to transforming our lifestyle so as to maximise our survivorship potential. The collective big picture can seem impossible to achieve and a little overwhelming. But by breaking this down into progressive smaller improvements – the metaphorical lifting of the bull – not only does reaching the desired goal suddenly appear achievable, but we feel motivated and inspired to strive for it in the realisation that small daily improvements consolidated over time really can reap staggering rewards. Our last focus needs to be on applying kaizen to the adoption of the survivorship practices we have explored all the way through this book in a strategic and practical way. To do so, I recommend my 5-Step Plan, which provides a clear roadmap for doing so.

## Step 1: Setting the Mind Up for the Exceptional

As we explored in chapters 3 and 4, our mind, and the emotions, beliefs, expectations and attitudes that flow through it, is the single most important tool we have for unleashing the deepest and most transformative levels of healing in the body. As such, your first priority needs to be setting up your mind for cultivating the genuine belief in your ability to become exceptional. To briefly recap, this centres upon:

# BRINGING IT ALL TOGETHER

- Embedding a daily meditation practice to neurologically increase the suggestibility of the brain in respect of the cultivation of such a belief.
- Protecting regular periods of contemplative time to develop clarity around your deepest and most meaningful goals, dreams and ambitions for the future.
- Creating immensely powerful imagery around the achievement of these goals.
- Harnessing the proven benefits of immune-stimulating guided imagery.

Your task in Step 1 is to explore these different practices and begin to embed them into your daily life in a slow but progressive manner using the concept of kaizen. For example, you might start with simply committing to a fifteen-minute meditation practice every day. Once that feels easy, you might extend this to twenty-five minutes and use the additional ten minutes to journal or explore your goals and dreams for the future in the way we discussed in chapter 4 (see Imagery Practice 2: Creating the Future Now – Goal-Setting Imagery on page 53). You might then extend this period of 'inner practice' by another ten minutes to allow you to embed a deeply powerful visualisation practice. By using kaizen in this way, you will, over time, develop a thirty-five-minute window every day to embed these foundational practices in a progressive, unintimidating and sustainable way. This may take a week or it might take several weeks, but don't progress to Step 2 until it intuitively feels like this step is flowing effortlessly. Then move on to the next step.

## Step 2: Supplying the Raw Materials of Exceptionality

The adoption of a robust anti-cancer diet informs a foundational practice within the overarching framework of cancer survivorship. Because of this, it is crucial that you begin the process of modifying and optimising your diet in keeping with the dietary evidence explored in chapter 5. However, as we have discussed, eating the correct types of anti-cancer food is only half of the dietary equation. You also need to proactively act in a way that allows for the full and complete digestion and assimilation of the nutrients within this food. To facilitate this, you should:

- Firstly, explore and begin to adopt the Recipes and Meal Plan found online at www.mind-body-medical.co.uk/becomingexceptional. This

will help to ensure that you are consuming meals that contain all of the six tastes of Ayurveda in a cancer-specific context, but with the help and guide of pre-formulated recipes, which initially makes things much easier.
- Before you go food shopping, spend time proactively planning your meals to ensure that you have the breadth of ingredients in your kitchen to allow for the daily adoption of the six tastes. This is particularly important when you move away from the provided meal plan and start constructing your own meals.
- Then commit to slowly transforming your diet until most of your meals comply with the nutritional advice provided in chapter 5.
- Remember the concept of kaizen here; you might just start by focusing on the modification and optimisation of your evening meal until doing so becomes effortless. At this point, expand your focus to also include your lunch and then your breakfast until all three of your daily meals are complying with the nutritional framework covered in chapter 5.
- Once this is flowing easily, turn to your digestion.
- Use the agni diagnostic guides in Understanding and Balancing Your Agni in chapter 6 (page 98) to assess the state of your agni right now. Having done so, commit to integrating a selection of the provided agni-balancing treatments to help bring increased balance to the workings of your digestive system.
- Commit to making these dietary and digestive goals your focus (while maintaining the previously embedded practices from Step 1) until they, too, become easy and habitual.
- At this point, look to progress to Step 3.

## Step 3: Herbal Empowerment

The next step is to begin the exploration and integration of anti-cancer herbal medicines into your survivorship protocol. As mentioned in chapter 7, it is vital that you do so in a completely safe and transparent manner. To facilitate this, physically action the following steps as the next target of your focus.

- Email or phone your clinical care team and schedule a meeting to explore the discussed herbs.
- Prior to this meeting, email your consultant the Memorial Sloan Kettering Cancer Center (MSKCC) weblinks for the recommended herbs

# BRINGING IT ALL TOGETHER

as discussed in chapter 7 (page 124) to allow them to read the clinical evidence around the herbs ahead of time. Also read up on these links yourself to allow for an informed and educated discussion around the use of the herbs as a supportive therapy to your conventional treatment plan.
- If your consultant is happy for you to start using the discussed herbs (which in my experience is around 70 per cent of the time), order and start using them as advised in Using These Herbs (page 134) in chapter 7. Please see Herbal Medicines (page 227) in appendix 3 for a list of the best suppliers to buy your herbs from.
- If a little more individualised support is needed, consider booking a consultation with a qualified medical herbalist or an Ayurvedic clinician.
- This step is an easy one in as much as almost no effort is required in terms of using and taking the herbal prescription; simply a minute or two of time each morning and evening.
- Once this step is underway, progress to Step 4.

## Step 4: Harnessing the Golden Hour and Dinacharya

Now comes arguably the biggest challenge and the one that requires the most concerted effort and commitment: embedding and harnessing the power of proper circadian alignment and adopting the Ayurvedic science of dinacharya (see Dinacharya on page 146). Of particular importance here is the establishment of the Ayurvedic optimal morning routine, which can truly transform the quality of your days. This undoubtedly requires significant levels of effort and self-motivation, and it is unquestionably hard at first. But it is also of vital importance beacuse the re-establishment of proper circadian alignment, and the embedding of the self-care practices contained within the prinicples of dinacharya, arguably represent some of the most powerful changes we can make in relation to healing. As always, we can apply the practice of kaizen to break down the overarching framework of dinacharya into achievable bite-sized pieces:

- Make the morning routine your initial priority; get this right and your energy, vitality and positivity will soar, as we saw in chapter 8 with the example of Liz's Experience of Brahma Muhurta on page 149.
- Commit to waking a little earlier to provide a protected period of time to progressively embed the morning routine practices we learned about

in chapter 8 – Embedding The Ayurvedic Optimal Morning Routine (page 151).
- Start with the practices that feel most important to you and make these your priority. For example, you may love how the practice of morning self-massage makes you feel. In which case, you might simply start by embedding that and nothing else.
- Once this is working well, you might then embed the journalling practices or the sun salutations.
- Use the concept of kaizen to continually progress your morning routine until you get it working in the best possible way for your specific circumstances.
- In the same way, continue to apply progressive change around the other key topics explored in chapter 8, most notably the circadian nutrition and evening routine practices.
- Action these steps slowly and progressively; don't rush or force them into your existing daily routine but let them unfold organically and naturally.
- Take heart from the fact that, each day, the changes you are making will get a little easier and soon they will become neurologically embedded in a way that will make them habitual and effortless. At such a time, move on to the fifth and final step.

## Step 5: Awakening Your Body's Inner Pharmacy

Last but by no means least, we turn to our final action step: awakening your body's inner pharmacy. I have purposefully left this step until last because it largely consists of practices that are quick and easy to implement, are in many cases passive (in that they require little time and effort to employ) and are typically perceived as being fun, and thus easy, to engage with. By saving them for last, we don't run the risk of over-burdening ourselves, given the effort already expended in the previous steps. The priority when actioning practices specific to awakening our inner pharmacy, as discussed in chapter 9, is *breadth*. In other words, it is better to spend a little time engaging a variety of different sensory practices than it is to spend more time on just one. This is because each practice engages and activates different physiological healing mechanisms and the more of these we activate the greater the collective benefit received. Here's some simple advice for doing so:

- Reread chapter 9 and make a list of the practices that intuitively appeal to you the most across the different senses.
- Then harness the ones that require virtually no active effort. For example, the next time you are sitting down to watch the television or to read, ensure an essential oil diffuser is active in the room. This will allow you to passively harness the profound healing benefits of essential oils without having to expend any energy doing so. Then perhaps create a beautiful collage or vision board of all the goals, dreams and holidays you want to experience over the coming year and gaze at this regularly.
- Once these practices are embedded, explore the feasibility and practicalities of forest bathing. I can't over-emphasise how important and transformative this can be and I strongly encourage you to make this a real self-care priority.
- Use the advice in How to Practise Forest Bathing in chapter 9 (page 183) to locate a forest bathing spot and commit to engaging the practices outlined on a regular basis.
- Lastly, you might explore the feasibility of booking a sensory retreat once or twice a year. You might spend time researching beautiful locations and finding remote cottages to stay in. You might decide to go on your own for a period of deep silence and solitude, or with loved ones. You might decide to go for a weekend or perhaps longer, but you go with the sole intention of immersing yourself in the type of sensory bubble explored in chapter 9. This is a hugely inspiring and motivating practice and one that creates real positive excitement and expectation for the future.
- As always, prioritise the concept of kaizen all the way through Step 5 to ensure small but continual progression rather than a singular drastic overhaul.

---

Over many years of employing these techniques and practices with thousands of people living with cancer, I have found that using a stepwise approach such as this is undoubtedly the most effective means of maximising long-term compliance. However, everyone's individual circumstances, motivation and level of health are different and it is important that you use the 5-Step approach purely as a general guide. If you feel motivated and that you would like to progress more quickly through the steps, then try adopting practices from different steps simultaneously. Conversely, if you are suffering with significant levels of fatigue or a heavy symptom load, it is important to conserve energy. In such situations you might choose to progress through the steps more slowly and focus on doing fewer practices until your overall levels of vitality increase. Furthermore, as you progress you must remain aware of the content explored in chapter 10 regarding the natural management of symptoms and side effects. The adoption of these holistic remedies, and the additional signposting resources recommended in this chapter, should be implemented in parallel to your progression through the five steps so that you can maintain the highest possible levels of health and vitality on a daily basis.

Through following the 5-Step Plan in this way, you have access to an all-encompassing blueprint for harnessing and unleashing the dynamic healing potential of the body via the integration of the timeless tradition of Ayurveda dovetailed with robust Western survivorship research. By marrying these two interdependent worlds together and integrating them into our daily lives using the progressive practices of kaizen, we do so in a way that works with the neurological mechanisms of the brain to promote compliance rather than non-compliance. And with that will always come profound transformation. Now it's over to you.

##  Chapter Affirmations for My Journey to Becoming Exceptional

1. I consciously acknowledge the inherent dynamism of my body and I recognise that I can harness this dynamism to in my quest to thrive in the face of cancer.
2. I consciously commit to providing my body, each and every day, with the correct types of raw material that it needs to harness this dynamism in the pursuit of transformational levels of healing.
3. I commit to using the practice of kaizen – implemented via the blueprint of the 5-Step Plan – to ensure the continual and progressive integration of the practices explored in this book in the knowledge that small daily improvements really can reap staggering rewards over time.
4. **Summary Affirmation:** Each and every day I commit to further strengthening my survivorship potential via the progressive application of the 5-Step Plan and the practice of kaizen.

# Conclusion

*Two men look out through the same bars; one sees the mud and one the stars.*

FREDERICK LANGRIDGE

Thousands of years ago, the towering Vedic philosopher and polymath Adi Shankara made a probing observation when he said, 'People get old and die only because they see other people get old and die.' He wasn't suggesting that ageing is an illusion and death avoidable. Rather, he was alluding to the power of negative association. More specifically, he was saying that, if what we observe always plays out the same way, it becomes impossible for us to see how it won't play out the same way for us too. In other words, the limits of our perception inform the limits of our reality.

The significance of this in relation to cancer survivorship is profound. Many years ago, I attended an integrative medicine conference in Milan. At one of the sessions, there was a German sociologist talking about how our perceptions of disease can shape the reality of it. She spoke about the fact that despite heart disease killing more people, and despite Alzheimer's disease being harder to manage, research shows that when large cohorts of people are asked which disease they most fear getting, the answer is almost always cancer. This opinion is not informed by fact; most of us are not aware of the up-to-date cancer prognoses data, the cancer treatment efficacy data or the most recent cancer survival statistics. Rather, it is informed by connotation.

Cancer is typically portrayed as being the scariest of diseases – the body turning against itself in a rampant and relentless process of self-destruction. Furthermore, cancer is a much more visual disease than most. We probably all know or have seen people who have lost their hair as a result of treatment, or who have lost lots of weight, or have been racked by nausea and vomiting. All these connotations conspire to make cancer appear incredibly scary. Which is correct: cancer *is* scary. But not more so than other life-threatening diseases. Catastrophic strokes, and the vegetative state they can leave us in, are equally scary. However, few people fear having a stroke in the same way they fear getting cancer. Looked at this way, the majority of the societal connotations inherent to cancer are unfounded. But the key point is that these connotations *will* go on to shape and colour our beliefs about cancer and, the more we subscribe to these beliefs, the greater the chance that they will become our reality.

Could this be what Shankara was alluding to? Could we paraphrase him and make the contentious statement: 'We deteriorate and die with cancer because we see others deteriorate and die with it'? It is my belief that there is a subtle element of truth to this. I am by no means implying that we can completely eradicate all cancer-induced suffering and death. It is not as simple as that. What I am suggesting is the all-pervading importance of moving beyond the limits of our vision to create a new reality around our ability to thrive and survive with cancer. More specifically, I would make the assumption that if one person – just one – has survived with the type of cancer you are living with, then theoretically others can too, including you. As such, it becomes imperative that we change the lens through which we formulate our deepest beliefs about cancer, for when we change how we look at things, the things we look at also change. And so, when we look at cancer through the lens of the exceptional cancer patient research, cancer itself takes on a different perspective. All sense of hopelessness and fear is blown apart, and in its place floods a genuine sense of optimism and hope around our ability to survive.

This concept brings me to the final point in this book and one that has ultimately underscored all of the content we have covered: the crucial need to have the courage to completely reperceive the notion of cancer in our lives and how we go about managing it.

Do we have the courage to stand up and initiate our move to becoming exceptional with the heartfelt conviction that we can achieve it?
Do we have the courage to perceive cancer as an opportunity?
Can we use it to help us live our lives more brightly, dream more powerfully and grasp every possible opportunity for love, awe and wonder in our daily lives?

Do we have the courage to free ourselves from the prison of our often limited vision and cultivate a genuine belief in our ability to regain our highest levels of health and wellbeing?

In my experience, these are prerequisites for becoming exceptional.

In writing this book, I have tried to create an alternate reality of cancer by reframing it as a disease that we have immense capacity to positively impact upon. And although we have now reached the end of this book, it is really just the start. Because now is the time to initiate *your* move into the exceptional. Now is the time to put in the hard work and actually do what needs to be done. I always think of the immortal words inspired by the poet Johann Wolfgang von Goethe when he said:

Whatever you can do, or dream you can, begin it; Boldness has genius, power and magic in it. Begin it now.

So begin. Dream big. Be daring. Laugh often. Love deeply and speak your truth. Cultivate excitement for the future. Work on yourself every day in a way that maximises your ability to become exceptional. And most importantly of all, sow the seeds of belief in your ability to survive and nourish them every single day until they bloom into an outlook of positivity that shapes and informs every facet of what makes you 'you'.

# Acknowledgements

Writing a book, I have discovered, is, perhaps more than anything else, a team effort, and I am so incredibly lucky to have the support of a truly amazing team, both professionally and personally.

To that end, I offer a heartfelt thank you to Muna Reyal, the head of editorial at Chelsea Green Publishing UK; it was her reaching out that ultimately led to the publication of this book and for that I am eternally grateful.

Likewise, I would like to thank the entire team at Chelsea Green Publishing for all of their help, support and encouragement throughout the whole process of publishing this book. And in particular to my editor, Susan Pegg, for all of her incredible help in getting the manuscript ready; I am grateful beyond words.

Over the last fifteen years, I have had the privilege of working with hundreds of unimaginably courageous people who have lived so brightly, positively and optimistically in the face of cancer. While you are too many to list individually, the impact you have had upon me is profound. You inspire me every day to live as brightly and as fully as possible and to help all those living with cancer who come after you to do likewise. Thank you.

Similarly, I would like to acknowledge Janet, the wonderfully courageous woman you met in the introduction to this book. As a close family member, I got to witness her journey to becoming exceptional from a much closer range than those I have worked with professionally. What I observed was a level of courage, self-belief and relentlessness that epitomised the very essence of what is needed move into the arena of exceptional. Janet, you still inspire me every single day and thank you for letting me be a part of your journey.

As someone living with dyslexia, proofreading has never been my strong point. As such, I owe a true debt of gratitude to those who were willing to help me in the proofreading of this book, namely Sue Hawkins, Saaria Alireza and my tireless mum, Gabby.

As mentioned in the introduction, I have been immensely fortunate to have crossed paths with two hugely influential mentors who have helped shape and influence my own beliefs and views around health and healing. To Dr Adrian Brito-Babapulle, a sincere thank you for introducing me to the wonders of natural medicine. And to Professor George Lewith, who sadly passed away several years ago, your views and beliefs around the limitless healing capacity of the body have now become my own, and I hope I can do both them and you justice in carrying this message forward.

To my amazing parents, to whom I owe everything. Without your unwavering support and help, I wouldn't be where I am today and for that I am truly grateful. You taught us to always strive to live the lives we want and to dream big, and I don't think there is any greater gift a parent can give their children, so thank you.

And lastly, to my own family. To my three children, Xavier, Trixie and Xanthe, and to my beautiful wife, Holly, I love you all beyond words; thank you for being you.

## APPENDIX ONE

# Vikruti Assessment Questionnaire

The following questionnaire has been designed to help you understand your current doshic make-up. This is your vikruti, which we learned about in chapter 2 under Ayurveda: The Science of Optimal Living on page 15. To complete the questionnaire, please think of how each statement applies to you as you are feeling right now. Answer by circling to what degree each statement applies to you, with 1 being the least and 6 the most. Please don't think too long or hard about each question; your first instinctive response will most likely be the accurate one.

### SCORING

Add up the collective scores for the twenty vata questions, the twenty pitta questions and the twenty kapha questions.

If one dosha is eight or more points higher than the other two, then that is your primary dosha.

If you have two doshas that are within eight points of each other, it means that you are dual-doshic. In this case, you will likely have strong characteristics of both doshas.

If all three doshas are within eight points of each other, then you are tri-doshic. This means you will likely have strong characteristics of each of the three doshas.

If you would like to learn more about the doshas, you can access my free online course Introduction to the Doshas at www.mind-body-medical.co.uk/becomingexceptional.

## Vata Dosha

1. I perform activity very quickly                              1 – 2 – 3 – 4 – 5 – 6
2. I am not good at memorising things
   and remembering them later                                   1 – 2 – 3 – 4 – 5 – 6
3. I am enthusiastic and vivacious by nature                    1 – 2 – 3 – 4 – 5 – 6
4. I have a thin physique – I don't gain weight easily          1 – 2 – 3 – 4 – 5 – 6
5. I learn new things easily                                    1 – 2 – 3 – 4 – 5 – 6
6. My characteristic walk is light and quick                    1 – 2 – 3 – 4 – 5 – 6
7. I tend to have difficulties making decisions                 1 – 2 – 3 – 4 – 5 – 6
8. I tend to develop gas or become constipated easily           1 – 2 – 3 – 4 – 5 – 6
9. I tend to have cold hands and feet                           1 – 2 – 3 – 4 – 5 – 6
10. I become anxious and worried frequently                     1 – 2 – 3 – 4 – 5 – 6
11. I don't tolerate cold weather as well as most people        1 – 2 – 3 – 4 – 5 – 6
12. I talk quickly and my friends think I am talkative          1 – 2 – 3 – 4 – 5 – 6
13. My moods change easily and I am emotional                   1 – 2 – 3 – 4 – 5 – 6
14. I often have difficulty in falling asleep and/or sleeping   1 – 2 – 3 – 4 – 5 – 6
15. My skin tends to be dry, particularly in winter             1 – 2 – 3 – 4 – 5 – 6
16. My mind is very active, restless and imaginative            1 – 2 – 3 – 4 – 5 – 6
17. My movements are quick and active;
    my energy comes in bursts                                   1 – 2 – 3 – 4 – 5 – 6
18. I am easily excitable                                       1 – 2 – 3 – 4 – 5 – 6
19. Left on my own my eating and sleeping habits
    become irregular                                            1 – 2 – 3 – 4 – 5 – 6
20. I learn quickly but also forget quickly                     1 – 2 – 3 – 4 – 5 – 6

## Pitta Dosha

1. I consider myself to be very efficient                       1 – 2 – 3 – 4 – 5 – 6
2. In my activities I am precise and orderly                    1 – 2 – 3 – 4 – 5 – 6
3. I am strong-minded and have a forceful manner                1 – 2 – 3 – 4 – 5 – 6
4. I feel uncomfortable and fatigued in hot weather             1 – 2 – 3 – 4 – 5 – 6
5. I perspire easily                                            1 – 2 – 3 – 4 – 5 – 6
6. Even though I don't always show it,
   I become angry/irritable easily                              1 – 2 – 3 – 4 – 5 – 6
7. If I skip a meal or delay eating,
   I become uncomfortable/angry                                 1 – 2 – 3 – 4 – 5 – 6

8. One or more of the following best describes my hair:
   early greying; balding; thin; fine; straight;
   blond, red or sandy coloured              1 – 2 – 3 – 4 – 5 – 6
9. I have a strong appetite and can eat a large quantity  1 – 2 – 3 – 4 – 5 – 6
10. Many people consider me stubborn         1 – 2 – 3 – 4 – 5 – 6
11. My bowel habits are regular              1 – 2 – 3 – 4 – 5 – 6
12. I become impatient very easily           1 – 2 – 3 – 4 – 5 – 6
13. I can be a perfectionist                 1 – 2 – 3 – 4 – 5 – 6
14. I get angry easily but then forget about it  1 – 2 – 3 – 4 – 5 – 6
15. I am fond of cold foods and cold drinks  1 – 2 – 3 – 4 – 5 – 6
16. I am more likely to feel a room is too hot than too cold  1 – 2 – 3 – 4 – 5 – 6
17. I don't tolerate foods that are hot and spicy  1 – 2 – 3 – 4 – 5 – 6
18. I am not tolerant of disagreement        1 – 2 – 3 – 4 – 5 – 6
19. I enjoy challenges and am very determined  1 – 2 – 3 – 4 – 5 – 6
20. I tend to be critical of myself and others  1 – 2 – 3 – 4 – 5 – 6

## Kapha Dosha

1. My natural tendency is to do things in
   a slow and relaxed way                    1 – 2 – 3 – 4 – 5 – 6
2. I gain weight more easily than most people
   and lose it more slowly                   1 – 2 – 3 – 4 – 5 – 6
3. I have a calm and placid disposition;
   people say I am 'chilled-out'             1 – 2 – 3 – 4 – 5 – 6
4. I can skip meals easily without any discomfort  1 – 2 – 3 – 4 – 5 – 6
5. I have a tendency towards excess mucus, phlegm,
   chronic congestion, asthma or sinus problems  1 – 2 – 3 – 4 – 5 – 6
6. I must get eight hours' sleep in order to be
   comfortable the next day                  1 – 2 – 3 – 4 – 5 – 6
7. I sleep very deeply                       1 – 2 – 3 – 4 – 5 – 6
8. I am calm by nature and not easily angered  1 – 2 – 3 – 4 – 5 – 6
9. I don't learn things as easily as some
   but have an excellent memory              1 – 2 – 3 – 4 – 5 – 6
10. I have a tendency to gain weight – I store fat easily  1 – 2 – 3 – 4 – 5 – 6
11. I dislike confrontation and like to maintain the peace  1 – 2 – 3 – 4 – 5 – 6
12. My hair is thick and wavy                1 – 2 – 3 – 4 – 5 – 6

13. I have smooth, soft skin                                       1 – 2 – 3 – 4 – 5 – 6
14. I have a large, solid body                                     1 – 2 – 3 – 4 – 5 – 6
15. The following describes me well:
    loving, affectionate, forgiving                                1 – 2 – 3 – 4 – 5 – 6
16. I have slow digestion, which often leaves me
    feeling heavy                                                  1 – 2 – 3 – 4 – 5 – 6
17. I have good stamina and a steady level of energy               1 – 2 – 3 – 4 – 5 – 6
18. I walk with a slow and measured gait                           1 – 2 – 3 – 4 – 5 – 6
19. I have a tendency towards over-sleeping,
    grogginess upon waking and I am slow
    to get going in the morning                                    1 – 2 – 3 – 4 – 5 – 6
20. I am a slow eater                                              1 – 2 – 3 – 4 – 5 – 6

## APPENDIX TWO

# Envisioning Health

### Guided Mental Imagery Script and Audio Download

The following is a detailed description of the immune-focused guided imagery script as explored in Imagery Practice 1: Envisioning Health in chapter 4 (page 51). To use this script, please read it through several times to familiarise yourself with it and to get a sense of how it works and what is required of you. Then you can read it aloud and record it to a cassette or digital dictation recorder, or to the voice notes on your phone, and then play it back to guide your practice. Alternatively, a free guided audio download of this imagery script can be accessed online at www.mind-body-medical.co.uk/becomingexceptional under Envisioning Health Guided Imagery.

1. You ideally want to complete this practice in a warm and relaxing room. Sit in a comfortable chair with your feet flat on the floor, your hands in your lap and your eyes closed.
2. Consciously let go of the day so far, and all of the demands placed upon you, and try to cultivate a sense of calmness and relaxation in your body.
3. Now, bring your awareness to your breath as it moves in and out of your body. In particular, hold your awareness on the movement of air as it flows in through your nostrils and down into your lungs. Focus on the expansion of your abdomen as you breathe and then its contraction as you breathe out, following the air as it moves up and out of your lungs via your nostrils.
4. Hold your focus on your breathing in this way for several minutes to help slow down the mind and induce a deeper sense of relaxation.
5. Now, before moving into the imagery practice, it is important to really induce a deeper sense of relaxation in the body, particularly the muscles. Doing so helps to remove any sense of stress or tension and further enhances the effectiveness of the subsequent imagery practice.

6. To do so, I would like you bring awareness to your toes. Tightly scrunch them together to create a palpable sense of tension. Then slowly release that tension as you uncurl them. Repeat this process once more and as you relax the toes the second time feel a deep sense of relaxation and heaviness in your feet.
7. Now, bring your awareness up into your calf muscles. To firstly create tension in these muscles gently lift your heels off the ground into a tiptoe position, feeling the tension in the calf muscles build as you do so. Then gently lower your heels back to the ground and as you do so feel the tension in the muscles melt away and a deep sense of relaxation flooding the lower leg area. Repeat this process a second time.
8. Continue to move your awareness up your legs and bring it to rest on the big muscles in your thighs. Gently squeeze your thighs together to create a palpable sense of tension in your thigh muscles. Hold that tension for a few seconds before relaxing the muscles, letting the legs fall open to experience a deep sense of relaxation in the big thigh muscles as you do so. Saviour the beautiful sense of heaviness in your legs as you feel the tension melt away. Repeat that process once again and then give both legs a gentle shake and acknowledge the heaviness and relaxation that lives there.
9. Next, move your awareness up to your shoulders and your neck. This is an area of the body that holds an immense amount of tension and stress and it's really important we remove that before engaging in practices such as guided imagery. To do so, gently but fully raise your shoulders all the way up to touch your earlobes as you breathe in, to create a real sense of tension in the shoulders and neck area. Hold that tension for a few seconds before gently lowering the shoulders, pulling them towards the floor as you exhale. Immerse yourself in the beautiful sense of relaxation and heaviness that accompanies that movement. Gently roll the shoulders forward and backwards once or twice before repeating the sequence again. Once you've done so, really acknowledge the sense of heaviness and relaxation in your shoulders and neck as you feel your body move into deeper full body relaxation.
10. Next, bring your awareness up to your face. Open your mouth as wide as it will go to create tension in the cheek and jaw muscles and hold that tension for a few seconds. Then gently shut your mouth and feel the tension in those muscles ebb away as you do so. Then bring your awareness to your eyes. Scrunch your eyes together to create real tension

in the muscles in and around the eyes and hold that tension for a few seconds. Again, release that tension as you experience a palpable sense of relaxation infusing your entire face.

11. Finally, let your awareness scan your whole body from the bottom of your feet to the top of your head, checking for any signs of tension, pain or discomfort. If you find any, gently breathe into that area and as you breathe out imagine the pain or tension dissipating as you experience a profound sense of relaxation across and within your entire body.

12. Having fully relaxed the body and mind, we now move into the imagery script. To do so, try to visualise in your mind either a symbolic or realistic image of the cancer you are living with. It is really important to think of the cancer as being very weak, confused and defenceless. Try to create an image of the cancer that reflects, in a profound way, these qualities of weakness and defencelessness. Also try to include details such as colour and shape. For example, a soft snowball melting under a hot sun implies a much greater level of weakness than a large rock in the same setting.

13. Next, move on to the creation of imagery of your immune cells, in either symbolic or realistic form. The quality, detail and accuracy of this immune-system imagery is of fundamental importance to the success of cancer-specific image practices. It is really important that the images you create depict immune cells that are immensely strong, undefeatable, highly aggressive and incredibly intelligent. Bring into your imagery the awareness of the all-conquering qualities of your immune cells; there is no contest between them and the cancer cells. When one of your immune cells comes into contact with a cancer cell, the immune cell will always win the battle and it is vital that the imagery you create around your immune cells depicts the inevitability of this.

14. Now visualise millions upon millions of these all-conquering immune cells flooding into the area of your body where the cancer exists. In the imagery you create, really try to induce a sense of this 'flooding-like movement' – this huge surge of super intelligent and immensely effective immune cells completely saturating the site of the cancer.

15. Next, slowly, and in as much progressive detail and accuracy as possible, see one individual immune cell select and then move towards one individual cancer cell. See them moving closer and closer together until they touch. See the immune cell, in whatever visual form it takes on in

your imagery, completely overwhelm the cancer cell before destroying it. As an example, you might imagine your cancer cell as a snowball and your immune cell as a huge blow torch. As the blow torch gets closer to the snowball, the inevitable melting and destruction of the snowball in unequivocal; there is no sense of this being a contest.

16. Next, increase the scale of this imagery to see the entire tumour melting away. Visualise the tumour mass getting smaller and smaller until not a trace remains. Visualise your immune cells surveying the scene one last time to check for any remaining rogue cells. Confident in the knowledge that none remain, visually scan the area where the tumour once was and, in your imagination, consciously acknowledge that there is no longer any cancer to be found there. Affirm to yourself that you are cancer free and that you will remain so for decades to come.

17. Now visualise yourself in the highest levels of health, vitality and well-being. Imagine yourself experiencing boundless levels of energy and see yourself engaging in normal daily activities – eating dinner with your loved ones, walking the dog, reading, cooking or shopping – from this place of vital, cancer-free health.

18. Give yourself a mental pat on the back to acknowledge all of the time, effort and motivation you are taking as you strive to move along the path to exceptional.

19. Before ending the practice, reaffirm to yourself out loud or silently in your head: 'I am cancer free, I will remain cancer free and every day in every way I am tirelessly moving into the realm of exceptional.'

20. Slowly open your eyes and reconnect with the room you are in. Finish by cultivating a massive smile before going out into the day.

N.B: Prior to actually practising this script, it can be tremendously helpful to firstly spend some time thinking about and visualising the images you will be using. Really think about how you perceive the cancer you are living with and what you imagine it to look like, in either real or symbolic form. The crucial point is that whatever imagery you decide upon, it must be perceived as being weak, vulnerable and confused. Once you have decided upon this, it can be really helpful to draw this image or find an image online that represents it. Then repeat this process for your immune cell imagery. With this decided upon, you are now best placed to actually engage in the practice.

# APPENDIX THREE

# Ayurvedic and Herbal Suppliers

## Herbal Medicines

**FUSHI**

Established in 2008, Fushi was founded with one purpose: to enhance people's wellbeing and inspire them towards happier, healthier lives using the wisdom of Ayurveda. They supply the very highest level of certified and organic herbal medicines, herbal oils, ghee and essential oils: www.fushi.co.uk.

**G. BALDWIN & CO.**

One of the oldest herbal apothecaries in Britian, Baldwin's offer a huge variety of herbal medicines, including all of those explored in this book: www.baldwins.co.uk.

**NAPIERS**

Another excellent source of herbal medicines and Scotland's oldest apothecary, Napiers stock a huge variety of herbs and they also offer free, qualified advice over the phone: www.napiers.net.

**ORGANIC HERB TRADING**

A leading supplier of organic medicinal herbs in the UK, they are more suited to buying herbs in bulk rather than in smaller volumes; however, they have an extensive range of herbs available: www.organicherbtrading.com.

**INDIGO HERBS**

An excellent supplier of all things herbal based in Glastonbury. They provide a wide selection of dried herbs and herbal powders, available in smaller volumes. They offer an excellent discount scheme: www.indigo-herbs.co.uk.

### BUY WHOLEFOODS ONLINE
A large distributor of both medicinal and culinary herbs with very competitive pricing. Trade accounts are available to further reduce costs: www.buywholefoodsonline.co.uk.

## Essential Oils and Sundries
### FUSHI
As well as supplying herbal medicines, Fushi also carry a large range of organic, top-quality essential oils: www.fushi.co.uk.

### TISSERAND
One of the oldest and most authentic manufacturers of essential oils, they also stock a wide range of relevant sundries, such as essential oil diffusers, pre-blended formulas, bath oils and much more: www.tisserand.com.

## Prebiotic, Probiotic and Synbiotic Supplements
### CHUCKLING GOAT
Producers of arguably the best-quality gut-health products in the world, I can't recommend Chuckling Goat enough. They provide the full range of prebiotic, probiotic and synbiotic supplements supported by free advice from their team of fully qualified nutritionists and gut health experts. They also offer comprehensive microbiome testing kits: www.chucklinggoat.co.uk.

## Ayurvedic Body and Massage Oils
### FUSHI
Fushi stock a wide variety of different herbal massage oils made using only the highest-quality ingredients: www.fushi.co.uk.

### ESSENTIAL AYURVEDA
An Ayurvedic-specific dispensary, they offer a good range of authentic Ayurvedic body and massage oils: www.essentialayurveda.co.uk.

# Glossary

**Abhyanga:** A specific type of Ayurvedic massage or self-massage.

**Agni:** Literally translating from the Sanskrit as 'fire', agni relates to the Western physiological understanding of the human gastrointestinal and digestive systems. Agni is responsible for the full and complete digestion and assimilation of the food we eat.

**Agni deepana:** The treatments used to bring balance and optimal functionality to the workings of agni.

**Ahamkara:** The subtle energy that ensures the harmonious workings of everything in the universe, including the human body. For example, it is ahamkara that allows an eye cell to support vision and a liver cell to support metabolism.

**Akashic field:** The conscious and intelligent primordial energy that existed in space and time before all matter in the physical universe was manifested in the Big Bang.

**Ama:** Dangerous and disease-forming toxic waste that builds up in the body, largely due to poor agni function, that goes on to disrupt the physiological workings of the body.

**Atman:** The Vedic concept of our soul or our innermost being that is beyond the realm of death or suffering; our true Self.

**Ayurveda:** Translated from the Sanskrit as 'the science of life', Ayurveda is a holistic system of medicine that originated in India around five thousand years ago. It has an unbroken lineage of use since that time and now has World Health Organization approval as a recognised system of medicine that supports the health of a large percentage of the world's population.

**Brahma muhurta:** Meaning 'the Creator's Time' in Sanskrit, Brahma muhurta refers to the early morning period before and after sunrise.

*Charaka Samhita:* The oldest and most revered clinical treatise in Ayurveda.

**Churna:** A pre-blended mix of culinary herbs that is added to cooking and seasoning as a way of optimising digestion.

**Dharma:** Dharma means 'the right way of living' and refers to the unique path we as individuals need to walk in life to ensure we bring meaning and purpose to our lives. Dharma also relates to the unique gifts and talents we were born with and how we honour these through our daily actions and decisions.

**Dinacharya:** Our daily routine and all of the self-care practices and behaviours we embed into our daily lives to maintain optimal health and wellbeing.

**Doshas:** The three doshas – vata, pitta and kapha – represent the unique mind-body constitutions of Ayurveda that inform how every facet of our bodies works and functions. They sit at the very centre of the Ayurvedic view of health preservation and disease management and allow for the individualisation of healthcare in a truly unique way.

**Kaizen:** A behavioural change practice based on the idea that small changes made daily are easier to adopt and comply with and thus induce greater gains.

**Kapha:** One of the three doshas, or mind-body constitutions, of Ayurveda.

**Manda agni:** A dysfunctional state of agni in the digestive system caused by a build-up of kapha.

**Mukta:** A state of consciousness that allows one to become fully liberated or freed from the sufferings of the mind and the body.

**Ojas:** Refers to the Ayurvedic understanding of immunity and protection. Ojas is also responsible for the provision of physical and emotional energy, vitality and vigour into our daily lives.

**Pilu agni:** The digestive process that allows nutrients circulating in the blood to cross the cell membrane and enter into our cells.

**Pitta:** One of the three doshas, or mind-body constitutions, of Ayurveda.

**Prakruti:** The unique doshic balance any given person was born with. This is fixed at the moment of conception and will remain unchanged for the duration of life. It represents the highest level of health and wellbeing.

**Rta:** The inner intelligence that exists as an inherent quality of every living thing and one that allows it to function and thrive in the most effective and harmonious way possible.

**Tanmatra chikitsa:** A specific framework of Ayurvedic healing using the senses.

**Tikshna agni:** A dysfunctional state of agni in the digestive system caused by a build-up of pitta.

**Turiya:** The fourth and highest state of consciousness, being above waking, sleeping and dreaming state.

**Vata:** One of the three doshas, or mind-body constitutions, of Ayurveda.

**Vikruti:** An imbalance in the doshas that is ultimately responsible for any ailments, diseases or problems experienced.

**Vishama:** A dysfunctional state of agni in the digestive system caused by a build-up of vata.

# Notes

**Chapter 2. Choosing Your Own Reality**
1. Maj-Britt Niemi, 'Cure in the Mind', *Scientific American Mind* 20, no. 1 (2009): 42.
2. Kelly A. Turner, *Radical Remission* (Bravo, 2015).
3. Candace B. Pert, *Molecules of Emotion* (Simon and Schuster, 1999).
4. Shirui Dai et al., 'Chronic Stress Promotes Cancer Development', *Frontiers in Oncology* 10 (2020), https://doi.org/10.3389/fonc.2020.01492.

**Chapter 3. The Biology of Hope – Unlocking the Gates of Exceptional**
1. Lissa Rankin, *Mind Over Medicine* (Hay House, 2021); David R. Hamilton, *How Your Mind Can Heal Your Body* (Hay House, 2008).
2. O. Carl Simonton, Stephanie Matthews-Simonton and James L. Creighton, *Getting Well Again* (Bantam, 1992).
3. Linda J. Luecken and Bruce E. Compas, 'Stress, Coping and Immune Function in Breast Cancer', *Annals of Behavioral Medicine* 24, no. 4 (2002): 336–344, https://doi.org/10.1207/S15324796ABM2404_10.
4. Jane T. Hickok, Joseph A. Roscoe and Gary R. Morrow, 'The Role of Patients' Expectations in the Development of Anticipatory Nausea Related to Chemotherapy for Cancer', *Journal of Pain and Symptom Management* 22, no. 4 (2001): 843–850, https://doi.org/10.1016/S0885-3924(01)00317-7.
5. Deepak Chopra and Rudolph E. Tanzi, *Super Brain* (Harmony, 2013).
6. Bruce Moseley et al., 'A Controlled Trial of Arthroscopic Surgery for Osteoarthritis of the Knee', *New England Journal of Medicine* 347, no. 2 (2002): 81–88, https://doi.org/10.1056/NEJMoa013259.
7. Brendan O'Regan and Caryle Hirshberg, *Spontaneous Remission* (Institute of Noetic Sciences, 1993).
8. Tim Lomas, Itai Ivtzan and Cynthia H.Y. Fu, 'A Systematic Review of the Neurophysiology of Mindfulness on EEG Oscillations', *Neuroscience & Biobehavioral Reviews* 57 (2015): 401–10, https://doi.org/10.1016/j.neubiorev.2015.09.018.
9. Michael Speca, Linda E. Carlson, Eileen Goodey and Maureen Angen, 'A Randomized, Wait-List Controlled Clinical Trial: The Effect of a Mindfulness Meditation-Based Stress Reduction Program on Mood and Symptoms of Stress in Cancer Outpatients', *Psychosomatic Medicine* 62, no. 5 (2000): 613–22, https://doi.org/10.1097/00006842-200009000-00004.
10. Linda Witek-Janusek et al., 'Effect of Mindfulness Based Stress Reduction on Immune Function, Quality of Life and Coping in Women with Newly Diagnosed Breast Cancer', *Brain, Behaviour and Immunology* 22, no.6 (2008): 969–81, https://doi.org/10.1016/j.bbi.2008.01.012.

**Chapter 4. Onwards to Imagery – The Recreation of Reality**
1. Denis Waitley, *The Psychology of Winning: Ten Qualities of a Total Winner* (Warner Books, 1986), 89.

2. Cecile A. Lengacher et al., 'Immune Responses to Guided Imagery During Breast Cancer Treatment', *Biological Research for Nursing* 9, no.3 (2008): 205–14, https://doi.org/10.1177/1099800407309374.
3. Angela K. Nooner, Kathleen Dwyer, Lise DeShea and Theresa P. Yeo, 'Using Relaxation and Guided Imagery to Address Pain, Fatigue, and Sleep Disturbances: A Pilot Study', *Clinical Journal of Oncology Nursing* 20, no. 5 (2016): 547–52, https://doi.org/10.1188/16.CJON.547-552.
4. O. Carl Simonton, Stephanie Matthews-Simonton and James L. Creighton, *Getting Well Again* (Bantam, 1992).
5. Barry L. Grubber, Nicholas R. Hall, Stephen P. Hersh and Patricia Dubois, 'Immune System and Psychological Changes in Metastatic Cancer Patients Using Relaxation and Guided Imagery: A Pilot Study', *Scandinavian Journal of Behaviour Therapy* 17, no. 1 (1988): 25–46, https://doi.org/10.1080/16506078809455814.
6. Shu-Fen Chen, Hsiu-Ho Wang, Hsing-Yu Yang and Ue-Lin Chung, 'Effect of Relaxation With Guided Imagery on the Physical and Psychological Symptoms of Breast Cancer Patients Undergoing Chemotherapy', *Iranian Red Crescent Medical Journal* 17, no. 11 (2015): e31277, https://doi.org/10.5812/ircmj.31277.
7. Deepak Chopra and Menas Kafatos, *You Are the Universe* (Rider, 2017).
8. Max Planck, *Scientific Autobiography and Other Papers* (Philosophical Library, 1968), 212.

## Chapter 5. Laying Strong Foundations – Ayurvedic Anti-Cancer Nutrition

1. Karen L. Chen et al., 'Impact of Diet and Nutrition on Cancer Hallmarks', *Journal of Cancer Prevention and Current Research* 7, no.4 (2017): 93–103, https://doi.org/10.15406/jcpcr.2017.07.00240.
2. Katrin Sak, 'Cytotoxicity of Dietary Flavonoids on Different Human Cancer Types', *Pharmacognosy Reviews* 8, no. 16 (2014): 122–46, https://doi.org/10.4103/0973-7847.134247.
3. Douglas Hanahan and Robert A. Weinberg, 'Hallmarks of Cancer: The Next Generation', *Cell* 144, no. 5 (2011): 646–74, https://doi.org/10.1016/j.cell.2011.02.013.
4. Claire M. Pfeffer and Amareshwar T.K. Singh, 'Apoptosis: A Target for Anticancer Therapy', *International Journal of Molecular Science* 19, no. 2 (2018): 448, https://doi.org/10.3390/ijms19020448.
5. Naghma Khan, Vaqar Mustafa Adhami and Hasan Mukhtar, 'Apoptosis by Dietary Agents for Prevention and Treatment of Cancer', *Biochemical Pharmacology* 76, no. 11 (2008): 1333–39, https://doi.org/10.1016/j.bcp.2008.07.015.
6. Dezhi Pan, Xue Gong, Xiaoqin Wang and Minhui Li, 'Role of Active Components of Medicinal Food in the Regulation of Angiogenesis', *Frontiers in Pharmacology* 22, no. 11 (2021), https://doi.org/10.3389/fphar.2020.594050.
7. Brendan O'Regan and Caryle Hirshberg, *Spontaneous Remission* (Institute of Noetic Sciences, 1993).
8. Yuexin Liu, 'Survival Correlation of Immune Response in Human Cancers', *Oncotarget* 3, no. 10 (2019): 6885–97, https://doi.org/10.18632/oncotarget.27360.
9. M.J. Proctor et al., 'The Relationship between the Presence and Site of Cancer, an Inflammation-Based Prognostic Score and Biochemical Parameters. Initial Results of the Glasgow Inflammation Outcome Study', *British Journal of Cancer* 103 (2010): 870–76, https://doi.org/10.1038/sj.bjc.6605855.
10. Yifeng Xia, Shen Shen and Inder M. Verma, 'NF-κB, an Active Player in Human Cancers', *Cancer Immunological Research* 2, no. 9 (2014): 823–830, https://doi.org/10.1158/2326-6066.CIR-14-0112.

11. Hany E. Marei et al., 'p53 Signaling in Cancer Progression and Therapy', *Cancer Cell International* 21 (2021): 703, https://doi.org/10.1186/s12935-021-02396-8.
12. Chen et al., 'Impact of Diet and Nutrition', 93–103.
13. Xiangming Guan, 'Cancer Metastases: Challenges and Opportunities', *Acta Pharmaceutica Sinica B* 5, no. 5 (2015): 402–18, https://doi.org/10.1016/j.apsb.2015.07.005.
14. Lara Saftić Martinović, Željka Peršurić and Krešimir Pavelić, 'Nutraceuticals and Metastasis Development', *Molecules* 25, no. 9 (2020): 2222, https://doi.org/10.3390/molecules25092222.
15. Kendra J. Royston and Trygve O. Tollefsbol, 'The Epigenetic Impact of Cruciferous Vegetables on Cancer Prevention', *Current Pharmacological Research* 1 (2015): 46–51, https://doi.org/10.1007/s40495-014-0003-9.
16. Ramesh Kumar Saini, Young-Soo Keum, Maria Daglia and Kannan R.R. Rengasamy, 'Dietary Carotenoids in Cancer Chemoprevention and Chemotherapy: A Review of Emerging Evidence', *Pharmacological Research* 157 (2020): 104830, https://doi.org/10.1016/j.phrs.2020.104830.
17. Laura L. Mignone et al., 'Dietary Carotenoids and the Risk of Invasive Breast Cancer', *International Journal of Cancer* 124, no.12 (2009): 2929–37, https://doi.org/10.1002/ijc.24334.
18. D. Ingram, 'Diet and Subsequent Survival in Women with Breast Cancer', *British Journal of Cancer* 69, (1994): 592–95, https://doi.org/10.1038/bjc.1994.108.
19. Onica LeGendre, Paul A.S. Breslin and David A. Foster, '(−)-Oleocanthal Rapidly and Selectively Induces Cancer Cell Death via Lysosomal Membrane Permeabilization', *Molecular Cell Oncology* 2, no. 4 (2015): e1006077, https://doi.org/10.1080/23723556.2015.1006077.
20. Ahmed Y. Elnagar, Paul W. Sylvester and Khalid A. El Sayed, '(−)-Oleocanthal as a c-Met Inhibitor for the Control of Metastatic Breast and Prostate Cancers', *Planta Medica* 77, no. 10 (2011): 1013–19, https://doi.org/10.1055/s-0030-1270724.
21. Grażyna Cichosz, Hanna Czeczot and Marika Bielecka, 'The Anticarcinogenic Potential of Milk Fat', *Annals of Agricultural and Environmental Medicine* 27, no. 4 (2020): 512–18, https://doi.org/10.26444/aaem/116095.
22. Abinaya Madhavan et al., 'Screening the Efficacy of Compounds from Ghee to Control Cancer: An In Silico Approach', *Biointerface Research in Applied Chemistry* 11, no. 6 (2021): 14115–26.
23. Hong-Wei Geng et al., 'Butyrate Suppresses Glucose Metabolism of Colorectal Cancer Cells via GPR109a-AKT Signaling Pathway and Enhances Chemotherapy', *Frontiers of Molecular Bioscience* 29, no. 8 (2021), https://doi.org/10.3389/fmolb.2021.634874.
24. Abdul Alim Bahrin et al., 'Cancer Protective Effects of Plums: A Systematic Review,' *Biomedicine and Pharmacotherapy* 146 (2022): 112568, https://doi.org/10.1016/j.biopha.2021.112568.
25. Nour Makarem et al., 'Consumption of Whole Grains and Cereal Fibre in Relation to Cancer Risk: A Systematic Review of Longitudinal Studies', *Nutritional Review* 74, no. 6 (2016): 353–373, https://doi.org/10.1093/nutrit/nuw003.
26. Mingsi Xie et al., 'Whole Grain Consumption for the Prevention and Treatment of Breast Cancer', *Nutrients* 11, no. 8 (2019): 1769, https://doi.org/10.3390/nu11081769.
27. Saray Gutiérrez, Sara L. Svahn and Maria E. Johansson, 'Effects of Omega-3 Fatty Acids on Immune Cells', *International Journal of Molecular Science* 20, no. 20, (2019): 5028, https://doi.org/10.3390/ijms20205028.
28. Raquel D. S. Freitas and Maria M. Campos, 'Protective Effects of Omega-3 Fatty Acids in Cancer-Related Complications', *Nutrients* 11, no. 5 (2019): 945, https://doi.org/10.3390/nu11050945.

29. C.J. Fabian, B.F. and S.D. Kimler, Hursting, 'Omega-3 Fatty Acids for Breast Cancer Prevention and Survivorship', *Breast Cancer Research* 4, 17, (2015) https://doi.org/10.1186/s13058-015-0571-6.
30. T. Liu et al., 'Molecular Mechanisms of Anti-cancer Bioactivities of Seaweed Polysaccharides', *Chinese Herbal Medicine* 13, no. 14 (2022), https://doi.org/10.1016/j.chmed.2022.02.003.
31. X. Lv et al., 'Citrus Fruits as a Treasure Trove of Active Natural Metabolites that Potentially Provide Benefits for Human Health', *Chem Cent J.* 24, no. 9 (2015), https://doi.org/10.1186/s13065-015-0145-9.
32. N. Clere et al., 'Anticancer Properties of Flavonoids: Roles in Various Stages of Carcinogenesis', *Cardiovasc Hematol Agents Med Chem.* 1, no. 9 (2011), https://doi.org/10.2174/187152511796196498.
33. A.S. Kristo, D. Klimis-Zacas and A.K. Sikalidis, 'Protective Role of Dietary Berries in Cancer', *Antioxidants* 19, no. 5 (2016), https://doi.org/10.3390/antiox5040037.
34. Aleksandra Kapała, Małgorzata Szlendak and Emilia Motacka, 'The Anti-Cancer Activity of Lycopene: A Systematic Review of Human and Animal Studies', *Nutrients* 14, no. 23 (2022), https://doi.org/10.3390/nu14235152.
35. A.P. Bhatt, M.R. Redinbo and S.J. Bultman, 'The role of the microbiome in cancer development and therapy', *CA: A Cancer Journal for Clinicians* 67, no. 4 (2017), https://doi.org/10.3322/caac.21398.
36. Ella Katz, Sophia Nisani and Daniel A. Chamovitz, 'Indole-3-carbinol: A Plant Hormone Combatting Cancer', *F1000Research* 1, no. 7 (2018), https://doi.org/10.12688/f1000research.14127.1.
37. S.V. Singh et al., 'Sulforaphane Inhibits Prostate Carcinogenesis and Pulmonary Metastasis in TRAMP Mice in Association with Increased Cytotoxicity of Natural Killer Cells', *Cancer Research* 69, no. 5 (2009), https://doi.org/10.1158/0008-5472.CAN-08-3502.
38. Gullanki Naga Venkata Charan Tej and Prasanta Kumar Nayak, 'Mechanistic considerations in chemotherapeutic activity of caffeine', *Biomedicine and Pharmacotherapy* 105 (2018), https://doi.org/10.1016/j.biopha.2018.05.144.
39. M.A. Martín, L. Goya and S. Ramos, 'Preventive Effects of Cocoa and Cocoa Antioxidants in Colon Cancer', *Diseases* 4, no. 1 (2016), https://doi.org/10.3390/diseases4010006.
40. Wolf Bat-Chen et al., 'Allicin Purified From Fresh Garlic Cloves Induces Apoptosis in Colon Cancer Cells Via Nrf2', *Nutrition and Cancer* 62, no. 7 (2010), https://doi.org/10.1080/01635581.2010.509837.
41. Jung Ok Ban et al., 'Inhibition of cell growth and induction of apoptosis via inactivation of NF-kappaB by a sulfurcompound isolated from garlic in human colon cancer cells', *Journal of Pharmacological Sciences* 104, no. 4 (2007), https://doi.org/10.1254/jphs.fp0070789.
42. Masood Sadiq Butt et al., 'Black pepper and health claims: a comprehensive treatise', *Critical Reviews in Food Science and Nutrition* 53, no. 9 (2013), https://doi.org/10.1080/10408398.2011.571799.
43. Azadeh Manayi et al., 'Piperine as a Potential Anti-cancer Agent: A Review on Preclinical Studies', *Current Medicinal Chemistry* 25, no. 37 (2018), https://doi.org/10.2174/0929867324666170523120656.
44. John F. Lechner and Gary D. Stoner, 'Gingers and Their Purified Components as Cancer Chemopreventative Agents', *Molecules* 24, no. 16, (2019), https://doi.org/10.3390/molecules24162859.

45. Tommaso Filippini, et al., 'Green Tea (*Camellia sinensis*) for the Prevention of Cancer', *The Cochrane Database of Systematic Reviews* 3, no. 3 (2020), https://doi.org/10.1002/14651858.CD005004.pub3.
46. Antonio Giordano and Giuseppina Tommonaro, 'Curcumin and Cancer', *Nutrients* 11, no. 10 (2019), https://doi.org/10.3390/nu11102376.
47. Irene Darmadi-Blackberry et al., 'Legumes: the most Important Dietary Predictor of Survival in Older People of Different Ethnicities', *Asia Pacific Journal of Clinical Nutrition* 13, no. 2 (2004): 217–20.
48. Shiwangni Rao et al., 'Inhibitory Effects of Pulse Bioactive Compounds on Cancer Development Pathways', *Diseases* 6, no. 3 (2018): 72, https://doi.org/10.3390/diseases6030072.
49. Hye-Jin Park, 'Current Uses of Mushrooms in Cancer Treatment and Their Anticancer Mechanisms', *International Journal of Molecular Sciences* 23, no. 18 (2022), https://doi.org/10.3390/ijms231810502.
50. Sahdeo Prasad et al., 'Recent Developments in Delivery, Bioavailability, Absorption and Metabolism of Curcumin: The Golden Pigment from Golden Spice', *Cancer Research and Treatment* 46, no. 1 (2014), https://doi.org/10.4143/crt.2014.46.1.2.
51. A. Ramesha et al., 'Chemoprevention of 7,12-dimethylbenz[a]anthracene-induced mammary carcinogenesis in rat by the combined actions of selenium, magnesium, ascorbic acid and retinyl acetate', *Japanese Journal of Cancer Research* 81, no. 12 (1990), https://doi.org/10.1111/j.1349-7006.1990.tb02685.x.

## Chapter 6. Agni and Ojas – The Elixir of Health and Immunity

1. S. Leviatan et al., 'An Expanded Reference Map of the Human Gut Microbiome Reveals Hundreds of Previously Unknown Species', *Nature Communications* 13 (2022): 3863, https://doi.org/10.1038/s41467-022-31502-1.
2. James Kinross, *Dark Matter* (Penguin Life, 2023).
3. S. Chandra, S.S. Sisodia and R.J. Vassar, 'The Gut Microbiome in Alzheimer's Disease: What We Know and What Remains to be explored', *Molecular Neurodegeneration* 18 (2023): 9, https://doi.org/10.1186/s13024-023-00595-7; Noor Akbar, et al., 'The role of gut microbiome in cancer genesis and cancer prevention', *Health Sciences Review* 2, (2022), https://doi.org/10.1016/j.hsr.2021.100010; M. Novakovic et al., 'Role of Gut Microbiota in Cardiovascular Diseases', *World Journal of Cardiology* 12, no. 4 (2020), https://doi.org/10.4330/wjc.v12.i4.110.
4. J. Durack and S.V. Lynch, 'The Gut Microbiome: Relationships with Disease and Opportunities for Therapy', *Journal of Experimental Medicine* 216, no. 1 (2019): 20–40, https://doi.org/10.1084/jem.20180448.
5. D. Zheng, T. Liwinski and E. Elinav, 'Interaction between microbiota and immunity in health and disease', *Cell Research* 30, (2020), https://doi.org/10.1038/s41422-020-0332-7.
6. Qiu Qin et al., 'Exploring the Emerging Role of the Gut Microbiota and Tumor Microenvironment in Cancer Immunotherapy' *Frontiers in Immunology* 11 (2021), https://doi.org/10.3389/fimmu.2020.612202.
7. Tomas Hrncir, 'Gut Microbiota Dysbiosis: Triggers, Consequences, Diagnostic and Therapeutic Options', *Microorganisms* 10, no. 3 (2022): 578, https://doi.org/10.3390/microorganisms10030578.
8. Iva Benešová, Ľudmila Křížová & Miloslav Kverka, 'Microbiota as the Unifying Factor behind the Hallmarks of Cancer', *Journal of Cancer Research and Clinical Oncology* 149 (2023): 14429–50, https://doi.org/10.1007/s00432-023-05244-6.

9. V. Srinivasan et al., 'Melatonin, Immune Function and Cancer', *Recent Patents on Endocrine, Metabolic and Immune Drug Discovery* 5, no. 2 (2011), https://doi.org/10.2174/187221411799015408.
10. Miroslav Pohanka, 'Impact of Melatonin on Immunity: A Review', *Open Medicine* 8, no. 4 (2013): 369–76, https://doi.org/10.2478/s11536-013-0177-2.
11. Masoud Moslehi et al., 'Modulation of the Immune System by Melatonin; Implications for Cancer Therapy', *International Immunopharmacology* 108 (2022): 108890, https://doi.org/10.1016/j.intimp.2022.108890.
12. J.R. Russel et al., 'Melatonin: A Mitochondrial Resident with a Diverse Skill Set', *Life Sciences* 301 (2022): 120612, https://doi.org/10.1016/j.lfs.2022.120612.
13. D. Dfarhud, M. Malmir and M. Khanahmadi, 'Happiness and Health: The Biological Factors- Systematic Review Article', *Iranian Journal of Public Health* 43, no. 11 (2014): 1468–77.

## Chapter 7. Nature's Pharmacy – Anti-Cancer Herbal Medicines

1. David J. Newman and Gordon M. Cragg, 'Natural Products as Sources of New Drugs over the Last 25 Years', *Journal of Natural Products* 70, no. 3 (2007), https://doi.org/10.1021/np068054v.
2. M. Ekor, 'The Growing Use of Herbal Medicines: Issues Relating to Adverse Reactions and Challenges in Monitoring Safety', *Frontiers in Pharmacology* 4, (2014), https://doi.org/10.3389/fphar.2013.00177.
3. B.B. Aggarwal, W. Yuan, S. Li and S.C. Gupta, 'Curcumin-free Turmeric Exhibits Anti-inflammatory and Anticancer Activities: Identification of Novel Components of Turmeric', *Molecular Nutrition and Food Research* 57, no. 9 (2013): 1509–1688, https://doi.org/10.1002/mnfr.201200838.
4. A.K. Chakravarty, S.N. Chatterjee, H. Yasmin and T. Mazumder, 'Comparison of Efficacy of Turmeric and Commercial Curcumin in Immunological Functions and Gene Regulation', *International Journal of Pharmacology* 5, no. 6 (2019): 333–45, https://doi.org/10.3923/ijp.2009.333.345.
5. Kelly A. Turner, *Radical Remission* (Barnet: Bravo Ltd, 2015).
6. Maryam Gul et al., 'Functional and Nutraceutical Significance of Amla: A Review', *Antioxidants* 11, no. 5 (2022): 816, https://doi.org/10.3390/antiox11050816.
7. Alok De et al., 'Sensitization of Carboplatinum- and Taxol-Resistant High-Grade Serous Ovarian Cancer Cells Carrying p53, BRCA1/2 Mutations by *Emblica officinalis* (Amla) via Multiple Targets', *Journal of Cancer* 11, no. 7 (2020):1927–39, https://doi.org/10.7150/jca.36919.
8. Sahitya K. Denduluri et al., 'Insulin-like Growth Factor (IGF) Signalling in Tumorigenesis and the Development of Cancer Drug Resistance', *Genes & Diseases* 2, no. 1 (2015): 13–25, https://doi.org/10.1016/j.gendis.2014.10.004.
9. Adele Chimento et al., 'The Involvement of Natural Polyphenols in Molecular Mechanisms Inducing Apoptosis in Tumor Cells: A Promising Adjuvant in Cancer Therapy', *International Journal of Molecular Science* 24, no. 2 (2023): 1680, https://doi.org/10.3390/ijms24021680; M.L. Rodríguez, J.M. Estrela and A.L. Ortega, 'Natural Polyphenols and Apoptosis Induction in Cancer Therapy', *Journal of Carcinogenesis & Mutagenesis* S6 (2013): 004, https://doi.org/10.4172/2157-2518.s6-004.
10. I. Singh, D. Soyal and P.K. Goyal, '*Emblica officinalis* (Linn.) Fruit Extract Provides Protection against Radiation-Induced Hematological and Biochemical Alterations in Mice', *Journal of Environmental Pathology, Toxicology and Oncology* 25, no. 4 (2006), https://doi.org/10.1615/jenvironpatholtoxicoloncol.v25.i4.40; R. Purena, R. Seth and R. Bhatt, 'Protective Role

of *Emblica officinalis* Hydro-ethanolic Leaf Extract in Cisplatin Induced Nephrotoxicity in Rats', *Toxicology Reports* 5 (2018): 270–77, https://doi.org/10.1016/j.toxrep.2018.01.008.

11. Tiejun Zhao, Qiang Sun, Maud Marques and Michael Witcher, 'Anticancer Properties of *Phyllanthus emblica* (Indian Gooseberry)', *Oxidative Medicine and Cellular Longevity* (2015): 950890, https://doi.org/10.1155/2015/950890.

12. Rajpreet Kaur Goraya and Usha Bajwa, 'Enhancing the Functional Properties and Nutritional Quality of Ice Cream with Processed *Amla* (Indian Gooseberry)', *Journal of Food Science and Technology* 52 (2015): 7861–71, https://doi.org/10.1007/s13197-015-1877-1.

13. Jasdeep Dhami, Edwin Chang and Sanjiv S. Gambhir, 'Withaferin A and Its Potential Role in Glioblastoma (GBM)', *Journal of Neuro-oncology* 131 (2017): 201–211, https://doi.org/10.1007/s11060-016-2303-x; Eun-Ryeong Hahm et al., 'A Comprehensive Review and Perspective on Anticancer Mechanisms of Withaferin A in Breast Cancer', *Cancer Prevention Research* 13, no. 9 (2020): 721–34, https://doi.org/10.1158/1940-6207.CAPR-20-0259; Nawab John Dar, Abid Hamid & Muzamil Ahmad, 'Pharmacologic Overview of *Withania somnifera*, The Indian Ginseng', *Cellular and Molecular Life Sciences* 72 (2015): 4445–50, https://doi.org/10.1007/s00018-015-2012-1; Peter T. White, Chitra Subramanian, Hashim F. Motiwala and Mark S. Cohen, 'Natural Withanolides in the Treatment of Chronic Diseases', in eds. S. Gupta, S. Prasad and B. Aggarwal, *Anti-inflammatory Nutraceuticals and Chronic Diseases, Advances in Experimental Medicine and Biology* 928, (Springer, 2016), 329–373, https://doi.org/10.1007/978-3-319-41334-1_14; In-Chul Lee and Bu Young Choi, 'Withaferin-A—A Natural Anticancer Agent with Pleitropic Mechanisms of Action', *International Journal of Molecular Sciences* 17, no. 3 (2016): 290, https://doi.org/10.3390/ijms17030290.

14. Y.K. Gupta, S.S. Sharma, K. Rai and C.K. Katiyar, 'Reversal of Paclitaxel Induced Neutropenia by Withania somnifera in Mice', *Indian Journal of Physiology and Pharmacology* 45, no. 2 (2001): 253–7.

15. B.M. Biswal et al., 'Effect of *Withania somnifera* (Ashwagandha) on the Development of Chemotherapy-induced Fatigue and Quality of Life in Breast Cancer Patients', *Integrative Cancer Therapies* 12, no. 4 (2013): 312–22, https://doi.org/10.1177/1534735412464551.

16. Aliya Sheik et al., 'The Anti-cancerous Activity of Adaptogenic Herb *Astragalus membranaceus*', *Phytomedicine* 91 (2021): 153698, https://doi.org/10.1016/j.phymed.2021.153698.

17. Mandy M.Y. Tin et al., '*Astragalus* Saponins Induce Growth Inhibition and Apoptosis in Human Colon Cancer Cells and Tumor Xenograft', *Carcinogenesis* 28, no. 6 (2007): 1347–1355, https://doi.org/10.1093/carcin/bgl238; K.K. Auyeung, P.K. Woo, P.C. Law and J.K. Ko, 'Astragalus Saponins Modulate Cell Invasiveness and Angiogenesis in Human Gastric Adenocarcinoma Cells' *Journal of Ethnopharmacology* 141, no. 2 (2012): 635–41, https://doi.org/10.1016/j.jep.2011.08.010.

18. Fanming Kong, Tianqi Chen, Xiaojiang Li and Yingjie Jia, 'The Current Application and Future Prospects of Astragalus Polysaccharide Combined With Cancer Immunotherapy: A Review', *Frontiers in Pharmacology* 12, (2021), https://doi.org/10.3389/fphar.2021.737674.

19. T. Fleischer et al., 'Improved Survival With Integration of Chinese Herbal Medicine Therapy in Patients With Acute Myeloid Leukemia: A Nationwide Population-Based Cohort Study', *Integrative Cancer Therapies* 16, no. 2 (2017): 156–64, https://doi.org/10.1177/1534735416664171.

20. Taixiang Wu, Alastair J Munro, Liu Guanjian and Guan Jian Liu, 'Chinese Medical Herbs for Chemotherapy Side Effects in Colorectal Cancer Patients', *Cochrane Database of Sysematict Reviews* 1 (2005), https://doi.org/10.1002/14651858.CD004540.pub2; Xue-Meng Pang

et al., 'Efficacy of Astragalus in the Treatment of Radiation-induced Lung Injury Based on Traditional Chinese Medicine: A Systematic Review and Meta-analysis of 25 RCTs', *Medicine* 101, no. 36 (2022): e30478, https://doi.org/10.1097/MD.0000000000030478.
21. D.T. Chu, W.L. Wong and G.M. Mavligit, 'Immunotherapy with Chinese Medicinal Herbs. II. Reversal of Cyclophosphamide-Induced Immune Suppression by Administration of Fractionated *Astragalus membranaceus* In Vivo', *Journal of Clinical and Laboratory Immunology* 25, no. 3 (1988): 125–9.
22. M.H. Chen et al., 'Integrative Medicine for Relief of Nausea and Vomiting in the Treatment of Colorectal Cancer Using Oxaliplatin-Based Chemotherapy: A Systematic Review and Meta-Analysis', *Phytotherapy Research* 30, no. 5 (2016): 741–53, https://doi.org/10.1002/ptr.5586.
23. Hong-Wen Chen et al., 'A Novel Infusible Botanically-Derived Drug, PG2, for Cancer-Related Fatigue: A Phase II Double-Blind, Randomized Placebo-Controlled Study', *Clinical and Investigative Medicine* 35, no. 1 (2012): E1–E11, https://doi.org/10.25011/cim.v35i1.16100.
24. Ping Wu, Jean Jacques Dugoua, Oghenowede Eyawo and Edward J. Mills, 'Traditional Chinese Medicines in the Treatment of Hepatocellular Cancers: A Systematic Review and Meta-analysis', *Journal of Experimental & Clinical Cancer Research* 28 (2009): 112, https://doi.org/10.1186/1756-9966-28-112.
25. S. Cheriyamundath et al., 'Aqueous extract of Triphala inhibits cancer cell proliferation through perturbation of microtubule assembly dynamics', *Biomed Pharmacother* 98 (2018), https://doi.org/10.1016/j.biopha.2017.12.022.
26. J. Tsering and X. Hu, 'Triphala Suppresses Growth and Migration of Human Gastric Carcinoma Cells *In Vitro* and in a Zebrafish Xenograft Model', *BioMed Research International* 10 (2018), https://doi.org/10.1155/2018/7046927.
27. Ramakrishna Vadde et al., 'Triphala Extract Suppresses Proliferation and Induces Apoptosis in Human Colon Cancer Stem Cells via Suppressing c-Myc/Cyclin D1 and Elevation of Bax/Bcl-2 Ratio', *BioMed Research International* 15 (2015), https://doi.org/10.1155/2015/649263.
28. Sahdeo Prasad and Sanjay K. Srivastava, 'Oxidative Stress and Cancer: Chemopreventive and Therapeutic Role of Triphala', *Antioxidants* 9, no. 72 (2020), https://doi.org/10.3390/antiox9010072.
29. Y. Zhao et al., 'An Integrated Study on the Antitumor Effect and Mechanism of Triphala Against Gynaecological Cancers Based on Network Pharmacological Prediction and In Vitro Experimental Validation', *Integrative Cancer Therapies* 17, no. 3 (2018), https://doi.org/10.1177/1534735418774410.
30. P. Belapurkar, P. Goyal and P. Tiwari-Barua, 'Immunomodulatory effects of Triphala and its individual constituents: a review', *Indian Journal Pharm Sci* 76, no. 6 (2014).
31. PDQ Integrative, Alternative, and Complementary Therapies Editorial Board 'Curcumin (Curcuma, Turmeric) and Cancer (PDQ®): Health Professional Version', *PDQ Cancer Information Summaries*, National Cancer Institute (US), 5 April 2024.
32. Atieh Ostadi et al., 'Therapeutic Effect of Turmeric on Radiodermatitis: A Systematic Review', *Physiological Reports* 11, no. 5 (2023): e15624, https://doi.org/10.14814/phy2.15624.
33. Masashi Kanai et al., 'A Phase I/II Study of Gemcitabine-Based Chemotherapy plus Curcumin for Patients with Gemcitabine-Resistant Pancreatic Cancer', *Cancer Chemotherapy and Pharmacology* 68 (2011): 157–64, https://doi.org/10.1007/s00280-010-1470-2; N. Martínez et al., 'A Combination of Hydroxytyrosol, Omega-3 Fatty Acids and Curcumin Improves Pain and Inflammation Among Early Stage Breast Cancer Patients

Receiving Adjuvant Hormonal Therapy: Results of a Pilot Study', *Clinical and Translational Oncology* 21 (2019): 489–98, https://doi.org/10.1007/s12094-018-1950-0.

34. Memorial Sloan Kettering Cancer Center, 'A Study Comparing a Plant-Based Diet with Supplements and Placebo in People with Monoclonal Gammopathy of Undetermined Significance or Smoldering Multiple Myeloma', last modified 15 February 2023, https://www.mskcc.org/cancer-care/clinical-trials/22-175.
35. S. Noreen et al., 'Pharmacological, nutraceutical, functional and therapeutic properties of fennel (*foeniculum vulgare*)', *International Journal of Food Properties* 26, no. 1 (2023), https://doi.org/10.1080/10942912.2023.2192436.
36. Hye-Jin Park, 'Current Uses of Mushrooms in Cancer Treatment and Their Anticancer Mechanisms', *International Journal of Molecular Sciences* 23, no. 18 (2022), https://doi.org/10.3390/ijms231810502.
37. Christine M. Kaefer and John A. Milner, 'The role of herbs and spices in cancer prevention', *The Journal of Nutritional Biochemistry* 19, no. 6 (2008), https://doi.org/10.1016/j.jnutbio.2007.11.003.

## Chapter 8. Dancing to Nature's Rhythm – Chronobiology and the New Frontier of Cancer Survivorship

38. W. Duan et al., 'Hyperglycemia, a neglected factor during cancer progression', *Biomed Res* 46 (2014), https://doi.org/10.1155/2014/461917.
39. V.P. Annamneedi et al. 'Cell Autonomous Circadian Systems and Their Relation to Inflammation', *Biomol Ther* 1, (2021) https://doi.org/10.4062/biomolther.2020.215.
40. Russell Foster, *Life Time* (Penguin Life, 2022).
41. R.C. Huang, 'The discoveries of molecular mechanisms for the circadian rhythm: The 2017 Nobel Prize in Physiology or Medicine', *Biomed J.* 41, no. 1 (2018), https://doi.org/10.1016/j.bj.2018.02.003.
42. C. Huang et al., 'Major roles of the circadian clock in cancer', *Cancer Biol Med* 12, no. 20 (2023), https://doi.org/10.20892/j.issn.2095-3941.2022.0474.
43. Tsuyoshi Oshima et al., 'Cell-based screen identifies a new potent and highly selective CK2 inhibitor for modulation of circadian rhythms and cancer cell growth', *Science Advanced* 5 (2019), https://doi.org/10.1126/sciadv.aau9060.
44. E. Cash et al., 'The role of the circadian clock in cancer hallmark acquisition and immune-based cancer therapeutics', *J Exp Clin Cancer Res* 40 no. 119 (2021), https://doi.org/10.1186/s13046-021-01919-5.
45. Y. Lee, 'Roles of circadian clocks in cancer pathogenesis and treatment' *Exp Mol Med* 53, (2021), https://doi.org/10.1038/s12276-021-00681-0.
46. K. Straif et al., 'Carcinogenicity of shift work, painting and fire fighting', *Lancet Oncology* 8, (2007), https://doi.org/10.1016/S1470-2045(07)70373-X.
47. J. Hansen, 'Night shift work and risk of breast cancer', *Curr Environ Health Rep* 4, no. 325 (2017), https://doi.org/10.1007/s40572-017-0155-y.
48. E. Filipski et al., 'Disruption of circadian coordination accelerates malignant growth in mice', *Pathol Biol* 51, 216 (2003), doi:10.1016/s0369-8114(03)00034-8.
49. B.J. Altman et al., 'MYC Disruption in the circadian clock and metabolism in cancer cells', *Cell Metabolism* 22, no. 6 (2015): 1009–19, https://doi.org/10.1016/j.cmet.2015.09.003.
50. Mark H. Rapaport et al., 'A Preliminary Study of the Effects of Repeated Massage on Hypothalamic–Pituitary–Adrenal and Immune Function in Healthy Individuals: A Study

of Mechanisms of Action and Dosage', *The Journal of Alternative and Complementary Medicine* 18, no. 8 (2012), https://doi.org/10.1089/acm.2011.0071.

51. C.C. Zouboulis, 'The skin as an endocrine organ', *Dermatoendocrinol* 1, no. 5 (2009), https://doi.org/10.4161/derm.1.5.9499.
52. L.B. Anna et al., 'A systematic review of gratitude interventions: Effects on physical health and health behaviors', *Journal of Psychosomatic Research* 135 (2020), https://doi.org/10.1016/j.jpsychores.2020.110165.
53. Alexandre Martchenko, Sarah E. Martchenko, Andrew D. Biancolin and Patricia L. Brubaker, 'Circadian Rhythms and the Gastrointestinal Tract: Relationship to Metabolism and Gut Hormones', *Endocrinology* 161, no. 12 (2020), https://doi.org/10.1210/endocr/bqaa167.
54. A.T. Hutchison, G.A. Wittert and L.K. Heilbronn, 'Matching Meals to Body Clocks—Impact on Weight and Glucose Metabolism', *Nutrients* 9, no. 3 (2017), https://doi.org/10.3390/nu9030222.
55. R. Klementand and M. Fink, 'Dietary and pharmacological modification of the insulin/IGF-1 system: exploiting the full repertoire against cancer', *Oncogenesis* 5, no. 193 (2016), https://doi.org/10.1038/oncsis.2016.
56. B. Gregory and G. Jamie, 'Biology of IGF-1: Its Interaction with Insulin in Health and Malignant States', *Novartis Foundation Symposium* 262 (2024).
57. K.L. Knutson et al., 'Role of sleep duration and quality in the risk and severity of type 2 diabetes mellitus' *Arch Intern Med* 166 (2006), https://doi.org/10.1001/archinte.166.16.1768; A. Malhotra and J. Loscalzo, 'Sleep and cardiovascular disease: an overview', *Prog Cardiovasc Dis* 51, no. 4 (2009), https://doi.org/10.1016/j.pcad.2008.10.004; E.N. Minakawa, K. Wada and Y. Nagai, 'Sleep Disturbance as a Potential Modifiable Risk Factor for Alzheimer's Disease', *International Journal of Molecular Sciences* 20, no. 4 (2019), https://doi.org/10.3390/ijms20040803.
58. Maria Paola Mogavero et al., 'Sleep disorders and cancer: State of the art and future perspectives', *Sleep Medicine Reviews* 56 (2021), https://doi.org/10.1016/j.smrv.2020.101409.
59. Kevin P. Collins et al., 'Sleep duration is associated with survival in advanced cancer patients', *Sleep Medicine* 32 (2017), https://doi.org/10.1016/j.sleep.2016.06.041.
60. Y. Li et al., 'Melatonin for the prevention and treatment of cancer', *Oncotarget* 13, no. 8 (2017), https://doi.org/10.18632/oncotarget.16379.
61. A. Büttner-Teleagă, Y-T. Kim, T. Osel and K. Richter, 'Sleep Disorders in Cancer—A Systematic Review' *International Journal of Environmental Research and Public Health* 18, no. 21 (2021), https://doi.org/10.3390/ijerph182111696.
62. Tara Sanft et al., 'NCCN Guidelines® Insights: Survivorship, Version 1.2023: Featured Updates to the NCCN Guidelines', *Journal of the National Comprehensive Cancer Network* 21, no. 8(2023), 792–803, https://doi.org/10.6004/jnccn.2023.0041.
63. J. Cipolla-Neto, 'Amaral FGD. Melatonin as a hormone: new physiological and clinical insights', *Endocrine Reviews* 39 (2018), https://doi.org/10.1210/er.2018-00084.
64. C.B. Swope et al., 'Factors associated with variability in the melatonin suppression response to light: A narrative review', *Chronobiology International* 40, no. 4 (2023), https://doi.org/10.1080/07420528.2023.2188091.
65. H.L. Rusch et al., 'The effect of mindfulness meditation on sleep quality: a systematic review and meta-analysis of randomized controlled trials', *Annals of the New York Academy of Sciences* 1445, no. 1 (2019): 5–6, https://doi.org/10.1111/nyas.13996.

## Chapter 9. Awakening the Body's Inner Pharmacy – The Sensory Pathways of Healing

1. Daisy Fancourt et al., 'The Psychoneuroimmunological Effects of Music: A Systematic Review and a New Model', *Brain, Behavior, and Immunity* 36 (2014), https://doi.org/10.1016/j.bbi.2013.10.014.
2. W. Thomas et al., 'Shamanism and Music Therapy: Ancient Healing Techniques in Modern Practice', *Music Therapy Perspectives* 7, no. 1 (1989), https://doi.org/10.1093/mtp/7.1.67.
3. Miyuki Suda et al., 'Emotional Responses to Music: Towards Scientific Perspectives on Music Therapy. *NeuroReport* 19, no. 1 (2008): 75–8, https://doi.org/10.1097/WNR.0b013e3282f3476f; Tamara L. Goldsby and Michael E. Goldsby. 'Eastern Integrative Medicine and Ancient Sound Healing Treatments for Stress: Recent Research Advances', *Integrative Medicine* 19, no. 6 (2020): 24–30.
4. Christopher Rennie, Dylan S. Irvine, Evan Huang and Jeffrey Huang, 'Music Therapy as a Form of Nonpharmacologic Pain Modulation in Patients with Cancer: A Systematic Review of the Current Literature', *Cancers* 14, no. 18, (2022), https://doi.org/10.3390/cancers14184416.
5. Margrethe Langer Bro et al., 'Kind of Blue: A Systematic Review and Meta-analysis of Music Interventions in Cancer Treatment', *Psychooncology* 27, no. 2 (2018), https://doi.org/10.1002/pon.4470; Russell E. Hilliard, 'The Effects of Music Therapy on the Quality and Length of Life of People Diagnosed with Terminal Cancer', *Journal of Music Therapy* 40, no. 2 (2003): 113–37, https://doi.org/10.1093/jmt/40.2.113.
6. Junling Gao, et al., 'The Neurophysiological Correlates of Religious Chanting', *Scientific Reports* 9 (2019): 4262, https://doi.org/10.1038/s41598-019-40200-w; Hazem Doufesh, Fatimah Ibrahim, Noor Azina Ismail and Wan Azman Wan Ahmad, 'Effect of Muslim Prayer (Salat) on α Electroencephalography and Its Relationship with Autonomic Nervous System Activity', *The Journal of Alternative and Complementary Medicine*. 20, no. 7 (2014): 558–62, https://doi.org/10.1089/acm.2013.0426.
7. Tsviya Olender, Doron Lancet and Daniel W. Nebert, 'Update on the Olfactory Receptor (OR) Gene Superfamily', *Human Genomics* 3 (2008):87, https://doi.org/10.1186/1479-7364-3-1-87.
8. A.M. Metwaly et al., 'Traditional ancient Egyptian medicine: A Review', *Saudi J Biol Sci* 28, no. 10 (2021), https://doi.org/10.1016/j.sjbs.2021.06.044.
9. Priyadaranjan Rây and Hirendra Nath Gupta, *Charaka Samhita: A Scientific Synopsis* (New Delhi: Indian National Science Academy, 1965).
10. John J. Steele 'The Anthropology of Smell and Scent in Ancient Egypt and South American Shamanism', in *Fragrance: The Psychology and Biology of Perfume*, eds. Charles S. Van Toller and G.H. Dodd (Elsevier Applied Science, 1992).
11. Dan Li et al., 'The Effects of Aromatherapy on Anxiety and Depression in People With Cancer: A Systematic Review and Meta-Analysis', *Frontiers in Public Health* 10 (2022), https://doi.org/10.3389/fpubh.2022.853056.
12. Hui Cheng et al., 'Aromatherapy with Single Essential Oils Can Significantly Improve the Sleep Quality of Cancer Patients: A Meta-Analysis', *BMC Complementary Medicine and Therapies* 22 (2022): 187, https://doi.org/10.1186/s12906-022-03668-0.
13. Lisa Demont, Amy Patterson, Tina M. Mason and Richard R. Reich, '99 – Complimentary Use of Essential Oils in the Autologous Blood and Marrow Transplant Population: Chemotherapy-Induced Nausea and Vomiting', *Transplantation and Cellular Therapy* 29, no. 2 (2023): S81, https://doi.org/10.1016/S2666-6367(23)00168-9.

14. Baraa A. L. Mansour, 'The Effect of Aromatherapy on Psychological Repercussions of Cancer Patients', *Zeugma Biological Science* 4 (2023): 1–6, https://doi.org/10.55549/zbs.872897.
15. Michihiro Nakayama, Atsutaka Okizaki and Koji Takahashi, 'A Randomized Controlled Trial for the Effectiveness of Aromatherapy in Decreasing Salivary Gland Damage following Radioactive Iodine Therapy for Differentiated Thyroid Cancer', *Biomed Research International* (2016), https://doi.org/10.1155/2016/9509810.
16. Fatouma Mohamed Abdoul-Latif et al., 'Exploring the Potent Anticancer Activity of Essential Oils and Their Bioactive Compounds: Mechanisms and Prospects for Future Cancer Therapy', *Pharmaceuticals* 16, no. 8 (2023), https://doi.org/10.3390/ph16081086; Mansi Sharma et al., 'Essential Oils as Anticancer Agents: Potential Role in Malignancies, Drug Delivery Mechanisms, and Immune System Enhancement', *Biomedicine & Pharmacotherapy* 146, (2022): 112514, https://doi.org/10.1016/j.biopha.2021.112514.
17. Richard Louv, *Last Child in the Woods* (Atlantic Books, 2010).
18. Anja Mehnert-Theuerkauf et al., 'Prevalence of Mental Disorders, Psychosocial Distress, and Perceived Need for Psychosocial Support in Cancer Patients and Their Relatives Stratified by Biopsychosocial Factors: Rationale, Study Design, and Methods of a Prospective Multi-center Observational Cohort Study (LUPE Study)', *Frontiers in Psychology* 14 (2023), https://doi.org/10.3389/fpsyg.2023.1125545.
19. Ye Wen, Qi Yan, Yangliu Pan, Xinren Gu and Yuanqiu Liu, 'Medical Empirical Research on Forest Bathing (*Shinrin-yoku*): A Systematic Review', *Environmental Health and Preventive Medicine* 24 (2019): 70, https://doi.org/10.1186/s12199-019-0822-8.
20. Qing Li, 'Effects of Forest Environment (Shinrin-yoku/Forest bathing) on Health Promotion and Disease Prevention – The Establishment of "Forest Medicine"', *Environmental Health and Preventive Medicine* 27 (2022): 43, https://doi.org/10.1265/ehpm.22-00160.
21. Josée Savard and Charles M. Morin, 'Insomnia in the Context of Cancer: A Review of a Neglected Problem', *Journal of Clinical Oncology* 19, no. 3 (2001), https://doi.org/10.1200/JCO.2001.19.3.895.
22. Claudia Trudel-Fitzgerald et al., 'Sleep and Survival Among Women with Breast Cancer: 30 Years of Follow-up within the Nurses' Health Study', *British Journal of Cancer* 116 (2017), https://doi.org/10.1038/bjc.2017.85.
23. Hyeyun Kim et al., 'An Exploratory Study on the Effects of Forest Therapy on Sleep Quality in Patients with Gastrointestinal Tract Cancers', *International Journal of Environmental Research and Public Health* 16, no. 14 (2019), https://doi.org/10.3390/ijerph16142449.
24. Bum-Jin Park et al., 'Effects of Forest Therapy on Health Promotion among Middle-Aged Women: Focusing on Physiological Indicators', *International Journal of Environmental Research and Public Health* 17, no. 12 (2020), https://doi.org/10.3390/ijerph17124348.
25. Qing Li, 'Effect of Forest Bathing Trips on Human Immune Function', *Environmental Health and Preventive Medicine* 15 (2010): 9–17, https://doi.org/10.1007/s12199-008-0068-3.
26. Jun-Shuai Xue et al., 'The Prognostic Value of Natural Killer Cells and Their Receptors/Ligands in Hepatocellular Carcinoma: A Systematic Review and Meta-Analysis', *Frontiers in Immunology* 13 (2022), https://doi.org/10.3389/fimmu.2022.872353.

## Chapter 10. Putting Out the Fires – Managing the Side Effects of Conventional Cancer Treatments

1. Edward B. Garon et al., 'Five-Year Overall Survival for Patients With Advanced Non-Small-Cell Lung Cancer Treated With Pembrolizumab: Results From the Phase I

# NOTES

KEyNOTE-001 Study', *Journal of Clinical Oncology* 37, no. 28 (2019), https://doi.org/10.1200/JCO.19.00934.

2. Peter Sonneveld et al., 'Daratumumab, Bortezomib, Lenalidomide, and Dexamethasone for Multiple Myeloma', *New England Journal of Medicine* 390, no. 4 (2024), https://doi.org/10.1056/NEJMoa2312054.

3. David Cella, Kimberly Davis, William Breitbart and Gregory Curt for the Fatigue Coalition, 'Cancer-Related Fatigue: Prevalence of Proposed Diagnostic Criteria in a United States Sample of Cancer Survivor', *Journal of Clinical Oncology* 19, no. 14 (2001): 3385–91, https://doi.org/10.1200/JCO.2001.19.14.3385.

4. Isa Hiske Mast et al., 'Potential Mechanisms Underlying the Effect of Walking Exercise on Cancer-Related Fatigue in Cancer Survivors', *Journal of Cancer Survivorship* (2024), https://doi.org/10.1007/s11764-024-01537-y.

5. Hsiang-Ping Huang et al., The Effect of a 12-Week Home-Based Walking Program on Reducing Fatigue in Women with Breast Cancer Undergoing Chemotherapy: A Randomized Controlled Study', *International Journal of Nursing Studies* 99 (2019): 103376, https://doi.org/10.1016/j.ijnurstu.2019.06.007.

6. Yasaman Khazaei et al., 'The Effects of Synbiotics Supplementation on Reducing Chemotherapy-Induced Side Effects in Women with Breast Cancer: A Randomized Placebo-Controlled Double-Blind Clinical Trial', *BMC Complementary Medicine and Therapies* 23, (2023): 339, https://doi.org/10.1186/s12906-023-04165-8.

7. Kun-Ming Rau et al., 'Management of Cancer-related Fatigue in Taiwan: An Evidence-Based Consensus for Screening, Assessment and Treatment', *Japanese Journal of Clinical Oncology* 53, no. 1 (2023), https://doi.org/10.1093/jjco/hyac164; Hong-Wen Chen et al., 'A Novel Infusible Botanically-Derived Drug, PG2, for Cancer-Related Fatigue: A Phase II Double-Blind, Randomized Placebo-Controlled Study', *Clinical and Investigative Medicine* 35, no. 1 (2012): E1–E11, https://doi.org/10.25011/cim.v35i1.16100.

8. PDQ Supportive and Palliative Care Editorial Board, 'Nausea and Vomiting Related to Cancer Treatment (PDQ®): Health Professional Version', *PDQ Cancer Information Summaries*, National Cancer Institute (US), 20 July 2023.

9. Zhenhua Jin et al., 'Ginger and Its Pungent Constituents Non-Competitively Inhibit Serotonin Currents on Visceral Afferent Neurons', *Korean Journal of Physiological Pharmacology* 18, no. 2 (2014): 149–53, https://doi.org/10.4196/kjpp.2014.18.2.149.

10. Julie L. Ryan et al., 'Ginger (Zingiber officinale) Reduces Acute Chemotherapy-Induced Nausea: A URCC CCOP Study of 576 Patients' *Support Care Cancer* 20 (2012): 1479–1489, https://doi.org/10.1007/s00520-011-1236-3.

11. Julie L. Ryan et al., 'Ginger for Chemotherapy-Related Nausea in Cancer Patients: A URCC CCOP Randomized, Double-Blind, Placebo-Controlled Clinical Trial of 644 Cancer Patients', *Journal of Clinical Oncology* 27, no. 15, (2009) https://doi.org/10.1007/s00520-011-1236-3.

12. Curlissa P. Mapp et al., 'Peppermint Oil: Evaluating Efficacy on Nausea in Patients Receiving Chemotherapy in the Ambulatory Setting', *Clinical Journal of Oncology Nursing* 24, no.2 (2020): 160–4, https://doi.org/10.1188/20.CJON.160-164.

13. Jean Toniolo, Valérie Delaide and Pascale Beloni, 'Effectiveness of Inhaled Aromatherapy on Chemotherapy-Induced Nausea and Vomiting: A Systematic Review', *Journal of Alternative and Complementary Medicine* 27, no. 12 (2021), https://doi.org/10.1089/acm.2021.0067.

14. A. Molassiotis, A.M. Helin, R. Dabbour and S. Hummerston, 'The Effects of P6 Acupressure in the Prophylaxis of Chemotherapy-related Nausea and Vomiting in Breast Cancer Patients', *Complementary Therapies in Medicine* 15, no. 1 (2007): 3–12, https://doi.org/10.1016/j.ctim.2006.07.005.
15. Ariah Bergman et al., 'Acceleration of Wound Healing by Topical Application of Honey. An Animal Model', *American Journal of Surgery* 145, no. 3 (1983): 374–6, https://doi.org/10.1016/0002-9610(83)90204-0.
16. Luyang Zhang et al., 'Use of Honey in the Management of Chemotherapy-Associated Oral Mucositis in Paediatric Patients', *Cancer Management Resources* 14 (2022): 2773–83, https://doi.org/10.2147/CMAR.S367472.
17. Chao Yang et al., 'Topical Application of Honey in the Management of Chemo/Radiotherapy-Induced Oral Mucositis: A Systematic Review and Network Meta-Analysis', *International Journal of Nursing Studies* 89, (2019): 80–87, https://doi.org/10.1016/j.ijnurstu.2018.08.007.
18. Tzu-Ming Liu et al., 'Prophylactic and Therapeutic Effects of Honey on Radiochemotherapy-Induced Mucositis: A Meta-Analysis of Randomized Controlled Trials', *Supportive Care Cancer* 27 (2019): 2361–2370. https://doi.org/10.1007/s00520-019-04722-3.
19. Ezgi Mutluay Yayla et al., 'Sage Tea–Thyme–Peppermint Hydrosol Oral Rinse Reduces Chemotherapy-Induced Oral Mucositis: A Randomized Controlled Pilot Study', *Complementary Therapies in Medicine* 27 (2016): 58–64, https://doi.org/10.1016/j.ctim.2016.05.010.
20. Ting Bao et al., 'Yoga for Chemotherapy-Induced Peripheral Neuropathy and Fall Risk: A Randomized Controlled Trial', *JNCI Cancer Spectrum* 4, no., 6, (2020): pkaa048, https://doi.org/10.1093/jncics/pkaa048.
21. Collette Mankowski et al., 'Effectiveness of the Capsaicin 8% Patch in the Management of Peripheral Neuropathic Pain in European Clinical Practice: The ASCEND Study', *BMC Neurology* 17, (2017): 80, https://doi.org/10.1186/s12883-017-0836-z.
22. Florent Bienfait et al., 'Evaluation of 8% Capsaicin Patches in Chemotherapy-Induced Peripheral Neuropathy: A Retrospective Study in a Comprehensive Cancer Centre', *Cancers* 15, no. 2 (2023): 349, https://doi.org/10.3390/cancers15020349.
23. B. Jordan et al., 'Systemic Anticancer Therapy-Induced Peripheral and Central Neurotoxicity: ESMO–EONS–EANO Clinical Practice Guidelines for Diagnosis, Prevention, Treatment and Follow-Up', *Annals of Oncology* 31, no. 10 (2020): 1306–19, https://doi.org/10.1016/j.annonc.2020.07.003.
24. TharatornTharatorn et al., 'Reduction in Severity of Radiation-Induced Dermatitis in Head and Neck Cancer Patients Treated with Topical Aloe vera Gel: A Randomized Multicenter Double-Blind Placebo-Controlled Trial', *European Journal of Oncology Nursing* 59 (2022): 102164, https://doi.org/10.1016/j.ejon.2022.102164; Pamela K. Ginex et al., 'Radiodermatitis in Patients with Cancer: Systematic Review and Meta-Analysis', *Oncology Nursing Forum* 47, no. 6 (2020): E225–E236, https://doi.org/10.1188/20.ONF.E225-E236.

# Index

Page numbers for glossary entries are in **bold**.

## A

Abhyanga 152–3, 195, **229**
acupressure 191–2
adenosine triphosphate (ATP) 115
*agni* 94, **229**
    as foundation of health 95–6
    and *ojas* building 113–14, 116
    synergy with gut microbiome 98
    understanding and balancing 98–113, 208
*agni deepana* 94, **229**
*ahamkara* (cellular consciousness) 21–4, **229**
    confusion and loss 22–3
    return 23–4
akashic field 55, **229**
Alexander the Great 129
Ali, Muhammad 10
alliums 85
aloe vera, topical 196
*ama* 97, **229**
American Cancer Society 48
amla (Indian gooseberry) 108, 127–9, 131
amygdala 176
anabolic ('sweet') taste 73–8
    angiogenesis 67
    drugs suppressing 67–8
    essential oils suppressing 177
    foods and nutrients suppressing 68, 73, 80, 81, 84, 86, 87, 88
    herbs suppressing 128, 130, 131, 133, 136
    and *ojas* building 117
    primary foods and anti-cancer actions 74–8
angiostatin 67
anthocyanins 76, 77
antioxidants 75, 80, 128, 129, 132
anxiety
    *Brahma muhurta* for 150–1
    cancer treatment-induced 170, 196–8
    forest bathing for 181
apoptosis (cell death) 23, 66–7
    essential oils inducing 177
    food and nutrients inducing 65, 67, 73, 75, 76, 77, 80, 81, 83, 84, 85, 86, 87, 88
    herbs inducing 131, 132, 133, 136
    meditation inducing 23–4
aromatherapy 176–8
ashwagandha (winter cherry) 129–30
astragalus (milk-vetch root) 130–1
    for cancer treatment-induced fatigue 189–90
astringent taste 86–9
*Atman* (consciousness, true Self, 'observer') 36, 38, **229**
    connecting with 36–7
Avastin 68
Ayurveda 6, 15–18, 121, **229**
    current medical paradigm compared 14
    and empowerment 3–4
    importance of diet 63
    inner pharmacy concept 169
    integrating with cancer survivorship research 5, 7, 23, 211
    integrating with conventional medicine 8
    *perfumeros* 177
    quantum theory compared 54–5
    restoration of balance 15
    river analogy 34
    role of mind in healing 26
    view and understanding of cancer 18–24
    *see also* six tastes of Ayurveda
Ayurvedic anti-cancer formulation 135
Ayurvedic chai 136–7
Ayurvedic circadian medicine *see dinacharya*
Ayurvedic evening routine *see* evening routine, Ayurvedic optimal
Ayurvedic herbs 8, 122–34
Ayurvedic kitchen herbal pharmacy 135–7

Ayurvedic morning routine *see* morning routine, Ayurvedic optimal
Ayurvedic oil self-massage *see* self-massage, Ayurvedic oil (self-abhyanga)

## B
Bannister, Roger 30–2, 34, 39
beliefs
    about healing foods 91–2
    importance in health and medicine 10–15
    Mr Wright's case 12–14, 17, 21
berries 80–1
beta brainwaves 38
bhibitaki 131
Big Bang 55
bitter taste 82–4
black pepper 85–6, 113
    synergy with turmeric 89
body
    awakening the inner pharmacy 165–86, 210–11
    continual change 34
    healing potential 5, 6, 202–5
*Brahma muhurta* (golden hour) 148–51, **229**
    Liz's experience 149–51
brain 20, 116, 212
    *Homo sapiens* 119
    impact of aromas 176, 179
    increasing suggestibility though meditation 38–40, 45, 207
    master clock (SCN) 143–4, 145, 149, 158, 162, 163–4
    *see also* frontal lobe; hypothalamus; neocortex dominance
brain cancer 145
brainwaves 35
    beta 38
    and sound therapy 170
    theta 35, 38, 39–40, 45
breakfast
    morning routine 156
    recipe 90
    timing 159
breast cancer 8, 58, 75, 128, 132, 179, 200
    foods and nutrients suppressing cancer hallmarks 74, 75, 77
    managing cancer treatment-induced side effect 130, 134, 188–9, 194
    meditation benefits 40
breath balancing 44–5
breath-based meditation 43
butyric acid 76

## C
C43 proteins 74
cancer
    Ayurveda and understanding of 18–24
    and circadian disruption 142, 145–6
    and gut microbiome 98
    herbal medicine research 121–2, 122–3
    meditation research 40–1
    reperceiving 213–15
    and stress 20
cancer cells 22–3
    imagining destruction 51, 52
    intellectualising to promote consciousness 23
cancer diagnosis, impact 9–10
cancer hallmarks 66, 127
    and anti-cancer nutrition 65–71
    home security system analogy 71
    practical applications of suppressing 71
    suppression through herbal medicine 126–34
    suppression through the six tastes of Ayurveda 72–91
cancer survivorship
    and aromatic medicine 177
    and circadian alignment 146
    and forest bathing 180–1
    and guided imagery 48–9
    impact of beliefs 12–14
    importance of diet 63–4, 64–5
    and melatonin 114
    and *ojas* building 113
    and perception of cancer 213
    and sleep dysfunction 161
    using herbal medicines safely 134
    *see also* exceptional cancer survivorship

# INDEX

cancer survivorship programmes 7
cancer survivorship research 6
    integrating Ayurveda 5, 7, 23, 212
cancer treatment side effects, managing 187–200, 212
    amla 128
    anxiety 170, 196–8
    ashwagandha 130
    astragalus 131
    essential oils 177
    fatigue 188–90
    impact of beliefs 28
    muscle aches and pains 195
    nausea and vomiting 190–2
    nerve pain/neuropathy 193–4
    oral mouth ulcers/mucositis 192–3
    radiotherapy-induced skin, mouth and throat discomfort 195–6
    support 198–200
    turmeric 134
capsaicin patches 194
carotenoids 74, 77, 81
cell contact inhibition 74
cells
    ability to think and express emotions 18–21, 23
    melatonin in 115
    nutrient delivery 93, 94
cellular clocks 144
cellular consciousness *see ahamkara*
cervical cancer 128
chanting 171–2
Charaka 131–2
*Charaka Samhita* 113, 121, 128, 131, 160, 177, **229**
chemotherapy *see* cancer treatment side effects, managing
chocolate, dark 84
churnas **229**
    kapha *agni*-balancing 111–12
    pitta *agni*-balancing 107
    vata *agni*-balancing 102–3
circadian alignment 144–5, 182
circadian cycle 140, 148
circadian disruption 141, 142, 145, 158

circadian medicine 141
circadian nutrition 157–60
    breakfast 159
    consistency 159–60
    dinner 159
    lunch 159
    12–3 model 159
    weight loss 160
circadian rhythm 142–6
citrus fruits 80
clinical settings, and music 172–3
coffee 83–4
colon
    gut microbiome 95
    toxicity 97–8
conjugated linoleic acid 75
consciousness
    cellular *see ahamkara*
    elevation 24
    fourth state (Atman, true Self) 35, 36–7, 38
    limitless potential 38
    *mukta* 26, **230**
    shift in, and recreation of reality 27–30
    three primary states 38
constipation 120
cortisol 143, 162, 173, 181
crucifers 83
curcumin 71, 87, 133
    from whole herbs vs isolated 123–5
cytokines 192

## D

Daratumumab 187
*dharma* 4, **229**
diet and nutrition 63–92, 207–8
    circadian nutrition 157–60
    hallmarks of cancer and anti-cancer nutrition 65–71
    importance of beliefs 91–2
    *ojas*-building foods 117
    practical application of suppressing the hallmarks of cancer 71
    six tastes of Ayurveda as anti-cancer nutritional blueprint 72–89
    using the six tastes in daily life 89–91

digestion 93–4, 207–8 *see also agni*
digoxin 122
*dinacharya* 142, 146–7, **229**
    what it is 147–8
dinner
    recipe 91
    timing 159
dopamine ('happy hormone') 116, 152, 170
*doshas* 15–18, 98, 177–8, **229**
    balancing 98–113, 175, 204
dysbiosis 97–8

### E
ego 37
Einstein, Albert 10, 33
empowerment 3–4
envisioning health imagery 51–3
    guided imagery script 223–6
    practice 52–3
    television analogy 52
epigallocatechin-3-gallate (EGCG) 71, 87
Epsom salt baths 195
essential oil diffusers 178, 191, 211
essential oils 176–7, 183
    for cancer treatment-induced nausea and vomiting 191
    using 177–8
European Society for Medical Oncology (ESMO) 194
evening routine, Ayurvedic optimal 160–4, 210
    avoid stimulation 162
    consistency in waking and sleeping 161–2
    meditation 163
    9 pm 'withdrawal' 163–4
    promoting *kapha* in the evening 162
    screen curfews 163
    sleeping environment 163
exceptional cancer survivorship
    and guided imagery 49–50
    and herbal medicine 126
    Janet's story 1–4, 54
    mechanism underpinning 21
    and *ojas* cultivation 116
    Penny's story 58–9
    and rebellious outlook 201–2
    research 5, 6–7, 14–15
    what Roger Bannister can teach us 30–6

### F
fatigue, cancer treatment-induced 188–90
fear 9
fermented foods 82
5-step plan 201–12
    step 1: setting the mind up for the exceptional 206–7
    step 2: supplying the raw materials of exceptionality 207–8
    step 3: herbal empowerment 208–9
    step 4: harnessing the golden hour and *dinacharya* 209–10
    step 5: awakening your body's inner pharmacy 210–11
flavonoids 80, 84, 128, 132
focus on five 155
forest bathing (*Shinrin-yoku*) 180–5, 211
    for cancer treatment-induced anxiety 198
    how to practice 183–5
    physiological and immunological benefits 182–3
    psychological and emotional benefits 181–2
foxgloves 122
Frankl, Victor 29–30
frontal lobe 51
    dominance 51–2

### G
Galen 48, 121
garlic 85
gastric (stomach) cancer 2, 132
Gayatri 172
geometric visual healing 175, 175 fig. 9.1
*Getting Well Again* (Simonton) 49
ghee 75–6
ginger 64, 86, 113
    for cancer treatment-induced nausea and vomiting 190–1
    phytocompounds 65, 72

# INDEX

ginger tea 86
gingerol 72, 190
goal-setting imagery 36, 53–62, 174
    Ayurveda, the unified field and quantum theory 54–8
    developing effective practice 60–2
    Penny's story 58–9, 61
    practising 58–9
Goethe, Johann Wolfgang von 215
golden hour *see Brahma muhurta*
gratitude 24, 154
green tea 87
Gregorian chants 172
growth inhibitors, evading 69–70
    aided by dysbiosis 98
    foods and nutrients and p53 reactivation 70
    and p53 gene mutation 69–70, 132
    triphala and p53 modulation 132
guided imagery 36, 47–62, 207
    envisioning health 51–3
    and exceptional cancer survival 49–50
    goal-setting imagery 53–62
gut microbiome 95–6
    butyric acid essential 76
    and cancer treatment side effects 189
    and colon toxicity 97
    and immune system 82, 96
    methods to support 96–7
    and probiotics 81–2
    relevance to cancer 98
    synergy with *agni* 98

## H

Hanahan, Douglas 66
haritaki 131
Hawking, Stephen 29
health behaviour change 204
hearing, sense of 167
    and forest bathing 184
    sound therapy 169–73
heart disease 122
herbal baths 197–8
herbal infusions and teas
    authentic Ayurvedic chai 137
    for cancer treatment-induced anxiety 196–7
    *kapha agni*-balancing 110–11
    *pitta agni*-balancing 106–7
    *vata agni*-balancing 101–2
herbal medicine 119–38, 208–9
    anti-cancer herbal pharmacy 126–34
    clinical investigation 121–2, 122–3
    herbs as medicine 122–6
    and human evolution 119–21
    *kapha agni*-balancing 112–13
    *pitta agni*-balancing 108
    polyherbal formulations 134
    safety 124–5, 126, 188, 208–9
    using 134–5
    *vata agni*-balancing 104
    whole herbs vs isolated compounds 123–6
herbal supplements 126
herbal synergy 134
herbs, culinary
    Ayurvedic kitchen herbal pharmacy 135–7
    *kapha agni*-balancing 112
    *pitta agni*-balancing 108
    *vata agni*-balancing 103
hing (asafoetida) 104
hippocampus 176
Hippocrates 48, 121
homeostasis (balance) 15, 26, 143
*Homo sapiens* 119, 175–6
honest reflection 154–5
honey, raw
    for cancer-treatment induced mucositis 192–3
    for radiotherapy-induced mouth and throat discomfort 196
hope 4, 21, 53–4
    biology of 25–46
human evolution
    and circadian disruption 140–1
    and use of herbal medicine 119–21
hummus 88, 91
hypothalamus 143, 149, 176

## I

immune activation, cancer-specific 68
    circadian medicine supporting 142

immune activation, cancer-specific (*continued*)
  foods and nutrients supporting 68, 74, 75–6, 77, 79, 82, 84, 85, 88, 87
  herbs supporting 128, 130, 131, 133
immune system
  activated by forest bathing 182–3
  communication with brain and nervous system 19–20
  enhanced by nature sounds 167
  envisioning health imagery 51–2
  and gut microbiome 82, 96
  impact of negative emotions 20
  impact of positive emotions 20–1
  and *ojas* 94, 115
  role of melatonin 115
  role of perforin 125
  suppressed by dysbiosis 98
  suppressed by stress 20
immunotherapy 187
indo-3-carbinoles 83
inflammation
  amla for 108
  forest bathing for 183
  healing aromas for 166
  healing sounds for 170
  herbal moth rinse for 193
  raw honey for 192, 196
  self-massage for 152
  and sleep dysfunction 161, 182
  topical aloe vera for 196
  turmeric for 134
inflammatory responses, cancer-mediated 68–9
  circadian medicine supressing 142
  foods and nutrients suppressing 69, 74, 77, 80–1, 83, 84, 85, 86, 87, 88
  herbs suppressing 108, 128, 130, 132, 133, 136
  increased by dysbiosis 98
  role of nuclear factor-kappa B (NF-κB) 69, 77, 85, 132
insulin growth factor-I (IGF-1) 128, 158
integrative cancer care 5, 6–8, 48–9, 50, 124, 177, 187, 212
integrative cancer charities 199–200

J
Jobs, Steve 201
journalling 154

K
*kaizen* 204–5, 207, 208, 209, 210, 211, **229**
  Hercules and the bull analogy 206
kale 73, 83
*kapha* 16, 98, 177, **229**
  evening promotion 162
*kapha* dominance 18
  essential oils for 178
*kapha*-imbalanced *agni* (*manda agni*) 109
  symptoms 109–10
  treating 110–13
Krebiozen 12, 13–14

L
*Last Child in the Woods* (Louv) 180
leafy green vegetables 83
leukaemia 131
Lewith, Professor George 7
limbic system 176
long pepper 113
lunar cycle 147, 160
lunch
  recipe 91
  timing 159
lung cancer 128
lycopene 81
lymphoma 12
lysosomes 75

M
Macmillan support services 198
Mahanarayan oil 195
*manda agni* (*kapha*-imbalanced *agni*) 109–13, **229**
Mandela, Nelson 29
matcha 87
Mayo Clinic, US 8, 48
meditation 6, 35, 36–8, 117
  and apoptosis 23–4
  balancing *doshas* 204
  breath balancing 44–5

breath-based 43
evening routine 163
increasing brain suggestibility 38–40, 45, 207
morning routine 153
practices 41–5
preparing for 41–2
psychological, emotional and physiological benefits 40–1
Vedic mantra 43–4
meditation space 42
melatonin
and dopamine regulation 116
immune-modulating activity 115
relationship to *ojas* 114–15
and sleep 144, 161, 162, 182
and synthesis of ATP 115
Memorial Sloan Kettering Cancer Center, US 8, 208–9
database 124
metastasis (invasion) 67, 70–1
essential oils suppressing 177
food and nutrients inhibiting 71, 75, 76, 77, 80, 81, 83, 86, 87, 88
herbs inhibiting 128, 130, 131, 133
mind
accessing latent power 35–6
impact on surgical healing 30
interpreting and recreating reality with 26–30
as matrix of matter 57
mental *vikruti* 17
potential for healing 25–6, 34
setting up for the exceptional 206–7
*see also* beliefs; negative mindset; positive mindset
mind-body practices 6, 7, 39, 49, 50
mind-over-matter 19
mineral salt 79
Minkowski vacuum 55
mission statement, author's 8
morning routine, Ayurvedic optimal 149, 150, 151–7, 209–10
Ayurvedic oil massage 152–3
breakfast 156–7

focus on five 155
gratitude 154
honest reflection 154–5
journalling 154
meditation 153
prayer 155–6
sun salutations 156
to-do list 155
waking up 151–2
mouth and throat discomfort, radiotherapy-induced 195–6
mucositis, cancer treatment-induced 192–3
*mukta* 26, **230**
muscle aches and pains, cancer treatment-induced 195
mushrooms 88–9, 136
music 172–3
myeloma 134, 149

## N

National Cancer Institute, US 190
National Comprehensive Cancer Network, UK 161
National Health Service (NHS), UK 7, 8, 58, 189
natural killer cells (NK cells) 40, 79, 82, 182
nature
and cancer treatment-induced side effects 198
sounds 167, 170–1
nausea and vomiting, cancer treatment-induced 190–2
negative feedback loops 26
negative mindset 6, 37–8
impact on immune system 20
Neiguan pressure point 191–2
neocortex dominance 37–8
calming through meditation 39–40
nerve pain/neuropathy, cancer treatment-induced 193–4
neuropeptide receptors 19
immune cells 19–20, 52
neuropeptides ('molecules of emotion') 19, 52
neuroplasticity 37

neuroreceptors 19
    olfactory 176
nocebo response 11–12
nuclear factor-kappa B (NF-κB) 69, 77, 85, 86, 132
nutrition *see* diet and nutrition
nutritional synergy 89–90
nuts and seeds 77–8

## O

observer effect 55–6
*ojas* 94, 113–18, **230**
    building robust 116–17
    and emotional health and vitality 116
    and immune system 94, 115
    *ojas*-building foods 117
    *ojas*-building lifestyle practices 117
    and physical energy, strength and vigour 115
    relationship to melatonin 114–15
oleocanthal 75
olfactory system 166, 176, 179
olive oil, extra-virgin 75
Olympic programme, US 47–8
om vibration 44, 170, 172
omega-3 fatty acids 77–8
one-to-one support 198–9
online cancer support forums 200
osteoarthritis 30
ovarian cancer 8, 128
oxygen atoms, and the body 203

## P

p53 gene ('guardian of the genome') 69–70, 132
    triphala modulation 132
pancreatic cancer 75
parasympathetic nervous system (PNS) 44–5, 167
particle and wave energy 55–6
peppermint essential oil 191
perforin 125
periphery clocks 144
Pert, Dr Candace 19, 21, 23
petrichor 179
pharmaceutical industry 122

phenolic compounds 76
phytochemicals 73, 83, 85, 87
phytocides 183, 184
phytocompounds 65, 83–4, 87
phytonutrients 66, 70, 74, 76, 80, 126, 128, 132, 133, 136
*pilu agni* 95, **230**
pink Himalayan salt 79
piperine 85–6
*pitta* 16, 98, 177, **230**
*pitta* dominance 18
    essential oils for 178
*pitta*-imbalanced *agni* (*tikshna agni*) 104–7
    symptoms 105–6
    treating 106–7
placebo response 11–12, 13–14
Planck, Max 57
plant-based medicines 122
plant-derived drugs 65
platelet-derived growth factor (PDGF) 69
polyphenols 84, 87, 128, 132
positive mindset 6, 9–10, 25–6, 215
    effect on immune system 20–1
potential quantum reality 56
*prakruti* 16, 26, **230**
    as hard wooden surface 17
prayer 155–6
prebiotics 189
probiotics 81–2, 189
proliferative growth signalling 70
    essential oils suppressing 177
    foods and nutrients suppressing 70, 74, 75, 76, 77, 79, 80, 81, 83, 84, 86, 87, 88
    herbs suppressing 130, 132, 133
prostate cancer 6, 75, 132
pulses 88
pungent taste 84–6

## Q

quantum theory 54–8

## R

*Radical Remission* (Turner) 14, 63
radiotherapy *see* cancer treatment side effects, managing

reality 25, 31, 35–6
    choosing your own 9–24
    creating a new around cancer 213–14, 215
    interpreting and recreating using mind 26–30
    recreating through imagery 47–62
    reshaping can change our body's healing response 34, 35 fig. 3.2
    reshaping can change the outcome 32, 33 fig. 3.1
    subjectivity of 27–8
root vegetables 74
ROS (reactive oxygen species) 132
*rta* 139–40, **230**

## S

sage, thyme and peppermint mouth rinse 193
salty taste 78–9
*sankalpa* 48
sea salt 79
seaweed 79
self-developing practices 153–6
self-fulfilling prophecies 11
self-massage, Ayurvedic oil (self-abhyanga) 152–3
    Mahanarayan oil 195
senna 120
sensory healing 165–86, 210–11
    forest bathing 180–5
    healing aromas 175–9
    healing images 173–5
    healing sounds 169–173
    senses and healing 166–9
sensory retreats 168, 211
serotonin 152, 170, 182
Shakespeare, William 29
shamans 121, 169
Shankara, Adi 213, 214
shatkona yantra hexagram 175, 175 fig. 9.1
sight, sense of
    and forest bathing 184–5
    healing images 173–5
Simonton, Dr O. Carl 48, 49–50, 51, 57–8
Simonton Cancer Center 49

six tastes of Ayurveda 64, 72–89, 208
    anabolic ('sweet') 73–8
    astringent 86–9
    bitter 82–4
    *kapha agni*-balancing 112
    *pitta agni*-balancing 107–8
    pungent 84–6
    salty 78–9
    sour 79–82
    *vata agni*-balancing 103
    using in daily life 89–91
skin discomfort, radiotherapy-induced 195–6
sleep 160–4, 204
sleep dysfunction 161
    forest bathing for 182
smell, sense of 166, 175–6
    essential oils 176–8
    and forest bathing 184
    Marion's experience 179
    other healing scents 178–9
soil and seed analogy 39
solar cycle 147
sounds *see* hearing, sense of
sour taste 79–82
stomach (gastric) cancer 2, 132
stone fruits, sweet 76
stress
    and cancer 20
    forest bathing for 181–2
sulforaphane 73
sulphur compounds 85
sun salutations 156
support for cancer treatment side effects 198–200
suprachiasmatic nucleus (SCN) 143–4, 145, 149
sympathetic nervous system (SNS) 44–5
synbiotics 189
synthetic drugs 123

## T

T-cells 75–6
table salt 78
*tanmatra chikitsa* 167, 168–9, 180, 183, 185, **230**
theta (healing) brainwaves 35, 38, 45
    and mind-body healing 39–40

*tikshna agni* (*pitta*-imbalanced *agni*)
  104–7, **230**
to-do list 155
Tom Baker Cancer Centre, Canada 40
tomatoes 81
Traditional Chinese Medicine (TCM) 130
trikatu 112–13
triphala 131–3
tulsi (holy basil) 104
*turiya* 38–9, **230**
turmeric (*jayanti*) 64, 87–8, 133–4
  synergy with black pepper 89
  whole herb vs isolated curcumin 123–5
12–3 model 159

## U
US Food and Drug Administration 13

## V
*vata* 16, 98, 177, **230**
*vata* dominance 18
  essential oils to balance 178
*vata*-imbalanced *agni* (*vishama*) 99–101
  treating 101–4
Vedas 169
Vedic mantra meditation 43–4
vibrational energy 55
*vikruti* 16–17, 23, **230**
  impact on *agni* 99
  as layer of dust 17
  mental 17
  removing 17, 204
Vikruti Assessment Questionnaire 18, 99,
  177–8, 219–22
*vishama* (*vata*-imbalanced *agni*) 99–104, **230**
vision boarding 24
vitamin C 128, 132

## W
Waitley, Denis 47–8
waking up 151–2
walking/aerobic exercise 188–9
weight loss 160
Weinberg, Robert 66
West, Dr Philip 12, 13, 14
wholegrains 76–7
Witek-Janusek, Linda 40
withanalides 129

## Y
Yes to Life, UK 199–200
yoga/Yogic practices 8, 24
  for cancer treatment-induced nerve
    pain/neuropathy 194
  sun salutations 156
yoga nidra 162

## Z
zingerone 190
zingiberene 72

# About the Author

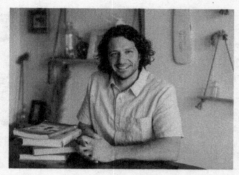
Julia Toms

Sam Watts has a PhD in cancer research from the University of Southampton's School of Medicine, where he worked for ten years. He has led large-scale NHS-funded cancer clinical trials in several leading hospitals, including Southampton General Hospital, Portsmouth's Queen Alexandra Hospital and University College London Hospitals NHS Foundation Trust.

Also a trained clinician of Ayurvedic and natural medicine, in 2018 Sam founded Mind-Body Medical to bring evidence-based and practical wisdom traditions of Ayurveda to those living in the UK and Europe. Mind-Body Medical has grown to become one of the leading providers of Ayurvedic healthcare in the UK.

Sam's passion lies in studying and exploring the clinical mechanisms that can empower those with cancer to become exceptional in terms of maximising the quality and quantity of life they experience. His research has been published in leading academic journals and he has presented at major integrative health and cancer conferences across Europe. In 2015, he was awarded the National Institute for Health Research (NIHR) Young Researcher of the Year award for research into prostate cancer survivorship.

the politics and practice of sustainable living
# CHELSEA GREEN PUBLISHING

Chelsea Green Publishing sees books as tools for effecting cultural change and seeks to empower citizens to participate in reclaiming our global commons and become its impassioned stewards. If you enjoyed reading *The Ayurvedic Approach to Cancer*, please consider these other great books related to integrative medicine and cancer.

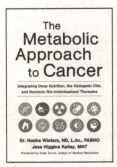

**THE METABOLIC APPROACH TO CANCER**
*Integrating Deep Nutrition, the Ketogenic Diet, and Nontoxic Bio-Individualized Therapies*
DR NASHA WINTERS AND JESS HIGGINS KELLEY
9781603586863
Hardcover

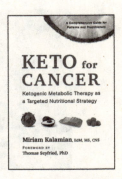

**KETO FOR CANCER**
*Ketogenic Metabolic Therapy as a Targeted Nutritional Strategy*
MIRIAM KALAMIAN
9781603587013
Paperback

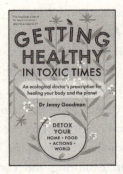

**GETTING HEALTHY IN TOXIC TIMES**
*An Ecological Doctor's Prescription for Healing Your Body and the Planet*
DR JENNY GOODMAN
9781915294333
Paperback

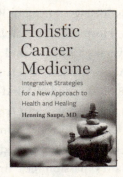

**HOLISTIC CANCER MEDICINE**
*Integrative Strategies for a New Approach to Health and Healing*
HENNING SAUPE, MD
9781645021551
Paperback

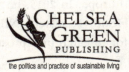

For more information,
visit www.chelseagreen.co.uk